# It Wasn't the Horse's Fault

## A Story of Hope, Hard Work, Love & Healing

Dear Elizabeth,

May this help you
understand a journey
we hope you never
have to take!

Doug
+
Pamela

"It Wasn't the Horse's Fault: A Story of Hope, Hard Work, Love, & Healing" Printed in the United States

Published by The Cheerful Word LLC

Cover design by Meghan McDonald

Cover art by Paula Poad

Joy of Spring by Brian Andreas 2016 used with permission

ISBN-10: 0-9978961-4-0
ISBN-13: 978-0-9978961-4-5

First printing, 2016

Additional copies can be ordered through www.amazon.com or at www.CheerfulWord.com

# Dedication

This book is dedicated to the thousands of
individuals who have, or will, face the tragedy
of suffering a severe brain injury.
To their families and friends, and to the
countless medical providers, therapists, and
caregivers who try to help them survive,
drive, and thrive.

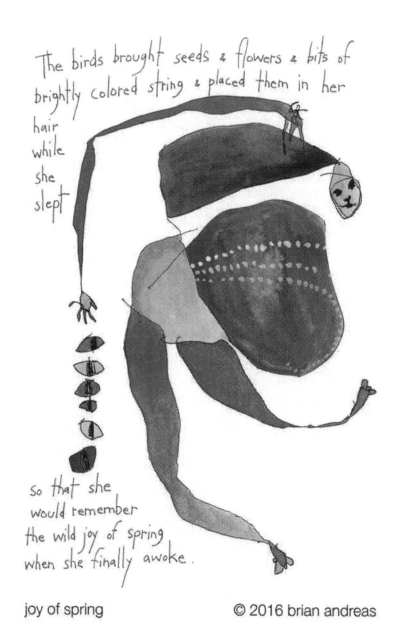

The birds brought seeds & flowers & bits of brightly colored string & placed them in her hair while she slept

So that she would remember the wild joy of spring when she finally awoke.

joy of spring

# Table of Contents

# TESTIMONIALS

*"I will never forget my time working with Paula and Doug. There are so many lessons from Paula and Doug's journey that I believe can help you find hope during the hardest times. This story is threaded with sadness, fear, unwavering love, hard work and perseverance, to achieve the best things in life acceptance and happiness. This family's journey was one of the best and most inspiring to me in my 15 years of being a physical therapist."*

Megan Burrowbridge Donaldson PT, PhD, FAAOMPT
Fellowship Trained Manual Physical Therapist
Associate Professor of Physical Therapy
Assistant Program Director of Physical Therapy, Walsh University

*"I have seen and treated hundreds of patients who have suffered head injuries, but not many who suffered one as severe as Paula had… and survived it. When I first saw her in the Emergency Room, I had no way of knowing how strong and stubborn she was and how much that would help her survive. I came to understand and appreciate the strength and drive in both Paula and her husband Doug in the days and weeks after my performing surgery to repair the*

damage caused by her fall from a horse. He knew that her injuries were life-threatening and extremely serious, but he seldom dwelt on that. Instead, he focused on learning everything he could about her condition and what was being done - and worked hard to be the support structure for her when she was incapacitated.

As a doctor, I seldom get the chance to follow patients' progress after they are discharged from my care, as there are always more patients in crisis that need my immediate attention. Doug and Paula are a team that I enjoyed following for years, through occasional visits and notes from them after they moved to another state. Their story is, indeed, one of hope, hard work, love, and healing. It can serve as an inspiration to others in the same situation and even those who appreciate that people facing incredibly life-changing events can survive, drive, and even thrive."

Georges Z. Markarian, M.D.

# PREFACE

I got to see her in the trauma room just before she was taken into surgery. The Paula I had breakfast with that morning wasn't there on that stretcher.

There were no outward signs of any serious injuries; she just looked like she was in a very deep sleep. But my best friend and wife had retreated to somewhere deep inside that complex, wonderful brain of hers. Someone handed me a plastic bag containing her earrings, necklace, and wedding ring they had to cut off her finger.

I remember thinking that we'd have a new one made when she got better. Then it hit me; she might not get better.

I'll never be able to erase the vision from my mind no matter how hard I try.

On a cool, beautiful, February day, all I can see is the blur of Boogie running away with Paula into the woods alongside Clypso with me astride. Both horses were spooked by the sudden start of an ATV nearby.

I watched in disbelief as Paula rolled off Boogie and disappeared on the other side of his body.

I pulled back on my reins so hard that they cut through the skin on a couple of my fingers. Clypso slid to a stop and I jumped off.

When I got to Paula lying on the ground, she was motionless. Her head had come to rest at the bottom of an oak tree with her neck bent at a ninety-degree angle. All the air was sucked out of my lungs when I saw that her eyes were only half open and that she was unconscious. I was sure she had broken her neck because I didn't think it could bend that far without breaking. I bent down to see if she was breathing. Thankfully, she was.

We've all heard the old saying that, "life can change in an instant." That is most certainly true, but it often takes much longer than that instant to appreciate how much life has actually changed and to learn how to live after it does.

Paula and I dealt with, and continue to cope with, the catastrophic change in our lives by focusing on three separate phases of life following her accident - surviving the initial accident, driving to recover as much of her former self as possible, and thriving in what might be called our "new normal." We found this to be the only way to cope with the initial crises and ongoing challenges we faced when our life-changing instant came along.

Our hope is that this book will inspire and encourage those who have experienced a severe traumatic brain injury, those who are caring for a loved one who has endured such an injury, and even those who know someone who has. We hope that our story gives health care professionals a better understanding of what their patients, who they care so much for, are going through.

Paula suffered a severe head injury. She was in a coma for about three weeks, couldn't move her right side or talk for almost a year and has had so many challenges after the injury that it's almost impossible to catalog them all.

We have included a number of pictures in this book that serve to highlight some of the important pieces of this journey. Some of them are graphic. These and other images I saw had an even greater impact on me than the pictures can convey. Some of these images and experiences are hard for me to describe and are the best way to show what we dealt with as Paula and I navigated this incredible journey together.

# Part One:

# Survive

Survive (ser-VAHYV): a verb, meaning to continue to live or exist, especially in spite of danger or hardship.

*"Courage is being afraid, but then doing what you have to do anyway."* Rudy Giuliani

First, we'll take you on a brief description of our life before the accident. Knowing who we were before she fell from the horse is an important part of understanding what happened and, more importantly, how we dealt with it.

We then take you with us through the journey that started in the woods behind our house as the paramedics worked on Paula. They took her to the nearest Level I trauma center, where teams of highly skilled and dedicated health care providers saved Paula's life and gave her the best opportunity to work on surviving her injuries.

After being in the Intensive Care Unit (ICU) in a coma for weeks, she gradually woke up and recovered to the point that she could be moved to an inpatient rehabilitation hospital. After a few weeks there, Paula crossed the line between surviving the accident and driving to recover her former self, which is where Part Two of our three-part book starts.

This book blends Paula's and my feelings, thoughts and experiences. Today, Paula doesn't remember much of anything about the accident, her time in ICU, and the first few days at HealthSouth in Monroeville, Pennsylvania, the rehab hospital she spent more than five months in after leaving the trauma hospital. For this reason, I provided most of the material for this chapter on surviving. As she began to wake up, which happened slowly - waking up from a coma does not happen in a moment's notice as is often portrayed in the movies - Paula started participating in life again and started to remember some of her experiences.

To help you understand who is speaking, Paula's feelings, thoughts, and experiences from before the accident and those after she started waking up again are shown in a different font throughout the book.

Winston Churchill is thought to have said, "When you're going through hell, keep going." Here are the first five months of Paula's ascension from hell in one montage.

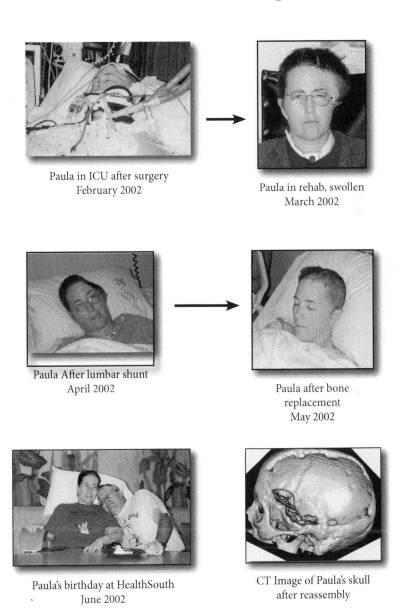

Paula in ICU after surgery
February 2002

Paula in rehab, swollen
March 2002

Paula After lumbar shunt
April 2002

Paula after bone
replacement
May 2002

Paula's birthday at HealthSouth
June 2002

CT Image of Paula's skull
after reassembly

It Wasn't the Horse's Fault

# CHAPTER 1

# LIFE AS WE KNEW IT: COLLEGE & THE NAVY

Paula and I were high school sweethearts. We went to different high schools in Sarasota, Florida and met during our senior year at a Winn Dixie grocery store where I worked after school. Paula shopped there for her family's groceries. We dated all through college. Paula graduated from the University of South Florida three months after I did. Two months after that, we pledged, among other things, to be with and support one another in sickness and in health as long as we both would live.

I worked for Allstate Insurance in St. Petersburg, Florida. After we got married, we moved into an apartment on the peninsula south of St. Petersburg. One Sunday, we were out driving around when we saw an open house in an old neighborhood near the center of the city. It was love at first sight, so we bought it from the eighty-year-old couple who owned it. They had been married for sixty years, which impressed us both.

About six months after we moved in, our next-door neighbors' daughter and her husband, a navy dentist with the rank of captain, were retiring from their last duty station in Keflavik, Iceland. They traveled to St. Petersburg to see her folks before settling down in their new home somewhere else. Her parents had us over for dinner and we listened in youthful excitement to their stories of traveling the world - seeing and doing so many interesting things during their twenty-five-plus years in the navy.

Later that night Paula asked me, "Have you ever thought about joining the navy?" I remember saying, "Not until tonight." We had tired of the Florida heat and Paula wasn't thrilled about living in Florida. I didn't see long-term potential in the job I held, so two weeks later, I was signed up to attend Officer Candidate School in Newport, Rhode Island. Paula's father was a retired Marine Corps officer and my brother was an Army Airborne Special Forces Ranger, so we knew a little about what we were getting into.

We put the house that we had lived in for less than a year on the market and made plans for some time apart while I was earning my commission as a Supply Corps ensign.

After a year and a half of training, including Officer Candidate School; Supply Corps School; and Submarine School, we were off to my first tour of duty on a ballistic missile submarine homeported in Charleston, South Carolina, and more than twenty-one years of excitement and fun travels with the navy. We lived in Detroit, Michigan; Groton, Connecticut; Lakehurst, New Jersey; Columbus,

Ohio; and even on the tropical Pacific Island of Guam. The navy even sent me to Pennsylvania State University to earn a master's degree in business administration.

We moved every three years or so. Paula worked a variety of jobs during my navy career including in picture frame shops, as a substitute teacher and teacher's aide, and as an aide in a group home for the disabled. Paula took on the responsibility for getting us ready for each move, helping us get through each move, and settling in each time. She saw to it that we were always ready to go for the next tour of duty.

Along the way, we traveled to some really cool places that we enjoyed thoroughly like Hawaii, Alaska, Bali, Singapore, Thailand, and Hong Kong.

We fell in love with traveling and put Paula's degree in cultural anthropology to good use. In Guam, she volunteered with the Officers' Spouses Club and worked in a bazaar they operated to raise money for a scholarship fund for military members' children. In this role, she got to go to some of those places mentioned earlier with $125,000 to spend on all sorts of stuff to be sold in the bazaar - talk about the ultimate shopping trip.

Paula bought Clypso, the first horse of our married life, near the end of our first tour of duty in Charleston. He was a beautiful two-and-a-half-year-old, saddlebred gelding. She owned him until he died at the age of twenty-seven and had confided to him things she never even told me. I'm perfectly okay with that because I understand the bonds of love that develop between women and their horses.

# Chapter 2

# A Deep & Abiding Love of Horses

Paula had horses for most of her life until she went off to college. In fact, her flea-bitten gray gelding, Sam, was there when I went to the barn to pick Paula up for our second date. He saw me as competition, pinned his ears back, and started to walk slowly in my direction. Even as a city slicker, I knew this was not a good thing and told Paula as much. She saw what was going on and told him that I was okay and to back off. Sam accepted me after that and Paula did, too.

I've always loved horses. The first time I got to ride by myself was at age five in Norfolk, Virginia. I rode a small pony that did a good job taking care of me. But one time he just wanted to be in the barn. So the pony, with me onboard, galloped back to the barn after jumping the ditch. I loved it. I think the adults were a bit upset.

We moved to Staunton, Virginia when I was around seven. We moved into an old house with a big barn and pasture and took two horses from the farm where we learned to ride in Norfolk. Mom started right away to get settled in the house.

My sister and I stayed out of the way. We had horses. That was enough. On my eighth birthday, I got a wonderful present: Candy, a pony. One I could ride by myself with no one else. So I started going farther and farther away from the older people. But not too far.

After riding her for a year, my mom knew I was too big for Candy. So when the horse trader showed up with a truck full of horses, she bought two of them. My father told him if he showed up again, he'd shoot him! Saber Dance was mine. He was about sixteen hands tall (about 64 inches at his shoulders) and a handful to ride, but a great horse.

My riding area grew. Jumping over jumps in our big field, riding through fields, woods, and dirt roads, and jumping fences after putting my coat on them to cover the wire—miles and miles to explore. Mom would drive around and try to find us if she thought we needed a rain coat or warmer coat. A lot of times, my girlfriend rode Candy and we'd go exploring. I didn't ride much in a ring. I'd just have a bridle on the horse and rode bareback. I was happy.

In 1969, my father fell and hurt his back. The doctors said he needed to avoid falling on ice or snow, so we moved down to Florida. All the horses stayed in Virginia. We lived in a subdivision with no horses!

My sister found a man who lived nearby. He had two horses that needed to be ridden. That helped with the need to be with horses. My mom, my sister, and I missed having horses. So after I ended the ninth grade, we moved again, out to a house in the country with a bit of land and a barn. My father was not happy with that, but he had three females that said we had to move and he lost. We got settled in and then got two horses. Jenny was my sister's. I got Sam, who was a good horse who went anywhere I asked him to go. He was careful to not step on me if I fell off.

During my senior year of high school, I met Doug. Doug and I went to different schools. He worked at the Winn Dixie where I shopped for groceries.

One day Doug saw me and asked a guy who he worked with that went to my school who I was. "Oh, her? That's Paula," he said. The guy told me the next day that a guy was asking about me. "What's his name?" "Doug Poad." I wondered how you spell Poad. A couple of days later my friend and I went grocery shopping. I went up to where Doug was working and asked him where the marshmallows were. He said they were out of season. That was the beginning of a good life together.

I remember one afternoon when I was out in the barn when Doug came in. He passed my horse, Sam. I looked up and saw Sam getting ready to make the new threat leave. I said, "Stop it, Sam! He's okay." He accepted him. Doug didn't ride, but he became a part of my life.

Then I graduated from high school. My mom and dad separated. We sold the house, Sam, and two other horses. I went off to a college in Virginia that had horses. I enjoyed that, but they only rode in a ring and I like trail rides in the woods. Plus I missed Doug. So I finished the next three years of college with him at USF. I found horses to rent while the three years went by. Back then you didn't have to ride with a leader. I'd just be out with a horse. Doug was always the love of my life, so after college, we got married. I didn't ride much for a while in our early married life together.

We were living in the city in St. Petersburg, Florida when Doug joined the navy and we moved out of Florida. I say he joined, but it was what we both wanted.

While he was off at Officer Candidate School, I lived with my sister in Virginia. She had a Morgan mare named Windy. We had to live in a trailer and find a place to keep Windy. I found a small field right near us, but I couldn't go for long rides. We were looking for a place she could buy that would have enough room to keep the horse there. I found it and we moved in. We had to put up fences and build a barn for her, but after that, Windy came home. I stayed with her while Doug completed Officer Candidate School and received his commission as an ensign.

After that, we moved to Athens, Georgia where he completed supply officer training. Then we moved to Connecticut, where he completed basic submarine training. I'd go down and see my sister when he was away. She had a filly named Mariah who was out of Windy's foal. The filly was neat to play with and hold in your lap.

The first sub he worked on was the USS Tecumseh. He'd be home for three months, then out for two and a half. When he was out to sea, I'd be up at my sister's. Near the end of him being out to sea one time, my sister decided she wanted to breed her Morgan mare with a saddlebred. She and I started looking at studs that would be what she wanted. One place we went to, she decided she didn't like the stud. The owner let the younger horses out to stretch their legs and one stole my heart. I asked the man if he had ridden him because he was about two. He said yes. I asked if he could show me how he was. So he put on his bridle and saddle and rode him around the arena. I asked how much he might want for him. The man said he wasn't good enough to be in shows, so he was cheap. I asked how much he would charge to haul him to my sister's.

Well, the horse was mine. I called him Clypso. When he got on the trailer there, it was the first time he'd ever been on a trailer. He got off at the end of the driveway at my sister's place and we walked him up the lane. He met my sister's horses over the fence and then naturally went in the field with them. He had a halter on and I walked him around the area. After a few days, I led him up to the fence and got on. He was still in a halter and lead line, no saddle or bit, but I rode him and all was fine.

Doug found out about him entering our life while he was underwater in the North Atlantic aboard his submarine.

I found out about it when my executive officer called me up to his stateroom to ask if I was expecting another family member. He had been given one of Paula's eight allotted twenty-eight word *familygrams* to me with the news that we had a new addition and he wanted to be the one to break it to me. He thought that I had forgotten to tell him before we left port that Paula was in the family way. I told him that it wasn't a two-legged addition and that I hoped it wasn't a horse.

Well, it was a horse, and it was a good thing that my specialty was logistics (making sure the right stuff is in the right place and knowing how to get it from point "A" to point "B"). We were living in South Carolina, Clypso was in Virginia, and we were moving to Michigan. Our only car was a Toyota Corolla station wagon. But it all worked out in the end.

Clypso lived in Michigan, Connecticut, New Jersey, Ohio, Virginia, Connecticut, and then back in Ohio again. We had to build barns and put up fences at almost all the places we moved. Doug and I enjoyed that. We had other horses come and live with us but we didn't buy and sell them. They just went to other places to live.

We moved Clypso to northeastern Ohio when we retired and Doug started teaching at Mount Union College. Clypso was getting older, so I thought of getting him a buddy. I started looking at horses for sale on the internet. One got my interest, a four-year-old saddlebred gelding named Tantoo that had never been ridden. I talked Doug into driving down to southern Ohio to see him.

I fell in love with Tantoo as soon as I saw him. My heart knew he should be with me so we bought him and changed his name to Boogie. It took a little while for Boogie and Clypso to accept one another and figure out who should rule the farm.

We put up a temporary round pen and a friend came over and started to gently teach Boogie how to be ridden. I got to be able to get on him after a while. After falling off three times, I discovered that riding Boogie without a saddle didn't work out too well. He didn't buck or shake, but I just couldn't stay with him, so he had to have a saddle, bridle, bit, and two reins. This was very different from riding Clypso, who I rode bareback with no bit. I rode Boogie around only in the field but I could ride Clypso with Boogie on a lead line right beside me. He'd happily walk, trot, and canter in the field, woods, or along the roads with no fear of anything.

# Chapter 3

# Life After the Navy

While at Penn State, I became convinced that my second career after leaving the navy should be teaching business in a small college. I taught evening classes at a local community college in New Jersey after earning my masters degree, and loved it. They liked me too, so it seemed like our future was set.

In 1998, about a year before I retired, I started pursuing a teaching career. I remember shouting to Paula from my home office one night that I had just found the job I wanted. A month before I retired in 1999, I signed a contract to start teaching that fall at Mount Union College in Alliance, Ohio, so it worked out pretty well. I settled into the new job with a great deal of satisfaction and determination. It was everything I'd hoped it would be and more.

In the late summer of 2000, just two years into my new dream job, two life-changing events took place.

First, I bought a brand new Chrysler PT Cruiser. I fell in love with it after seeing pictures of it online at the Detroit Auto Show. I did a little research on it and ordered one without having ever seen one, let alone taking one for a test drive. Mine was only the second one delivered in the whole county. I put subdued flames on the sides, got a vanity plate that read POADSTER, washed and waxed it once or twice a week. I became part of a large group of middle-aged folks who somehow saw it, at least subconsciously, as a connection to our youth. In some sort of weird midlife crisis, I even put a glass pack muffler on it to enjoy that deep, rumbling exhaust sound that I remember liking in my teens. It didn't end up being nearly as enjoyable as the ones in my teens, but more on that later.

Second, Paula fell in love on the internet, too. I was in my home office grading some papers and she called for me to come see something on her computer. Turns out there was a horse for sale about one hundred miles south of us in southern Ohio. He was a four-year-old, saddlebred gelding named Tantoo. She said that she wanted to go see him. I recall asking if we needed another horse. Then I think I asked if we should take the horse trailer. Paula fell in love immediately.

We brought him home and changed his name to Boogie. Boogie had not been ridden much. He was hard to train for riding because he had been in a stall for most of his life. He wasn't a mean horse, but he was a handful. Since he was only green broke, we put a round pen in the back pasture and she commenced his training.

A friend who trained horses helped her at first, but soon she was working him on her own in the pen. I remember seeing and hearing her falling off in the round pen several times during his training. She also took him out on rides with her and Clypso, Boogie trailing along behind them on a lead line or, as Paula called it, being ponied.

In a few months, she could ride him around the round pen with a saddle, bridle, bit, and reins. She often rode Clypso with only a bathroom rug to sit on and a piece of baling twine around his neck for reins, so this was more tack than she normally used.

# CHAPTER 4

# CHANGE IN PLANS

With my navy retirement income and health care giving us a decent foundation, we intended to spend a good deal of my salary from teaching on plane tickets and hotel rooms to travel to lots of places we hadn't seen yet, and also some places that we wanted to see again like Bali and northern Thailand.

We tend to do special things on what we call our speed-limit anniversaries (i.e. 15, 20, 25, etc.). For our twentieth anniversary in 1996, we took a fifteen-day trip to Hong Kong and Thailand. On that special day of our anniversary, we were riding elephants in northern Thailand.

For our twenty-fifth anniversary in 2001, we flew to Alaska for fifteen days, rented a car, and saw just about every mile of paved highway outside the big cities.

Meanwhile, I was thriving at Mount Union; enjoying it very much and making some real positive contributions to the college and students. Life was playing out pretty much as we had planned and we were enjoying every minute of it.

February 9, 2002 was a Saturday. It dawned bright and clear in northeastern Ohio. The weather forecast was for unseasonably warm weather, around forty-five degrees. It was a day made for being outside.

I didn't ride very often—not nearly as much as Paula would have liked—but I knew that Paula wanted to go riding and that she wanted me to tag along. It wouldn't be warmer until mid-afternoon, so we did a few things in the morning before heading out.

I removed that noisy muffler on the PT Cruiser and replaced it with a standard stock muffler. After I got the muffler replaced, we went for a ride to see how it sounded.

While we were out, we went to look at a couple of donkeys that a man nearby had for sale. We weren't really in the market for a donkey. Clypso and Boogie already had each other for company. Going to see the donkeys was more of a curiosity than a plan. We did talk about having a donkey to keep the coyotes off our land. Donkeys seem to hate coyotes and will actually kill them if they get the chance. Coyotes weren't a major problem, but we did have cats that went outside, so we weren't exactly not in the market for one, either.

I wish we had bought one because it may have saved us from what was to come that day.

We returned home without a donkey and Paula wanted me to go riding with her. I only rode once or twice a year because I would rather play golf. Paula said to me, "You know, we're not going to have many days like this until spring, so let's go riding." So I agreed and changed clothes. Our two dogs were excited about going for a ride, too.

In the early afternoon warmth, we saddled up the horses and rode through our neighbor's yard, following an old trail into the woods behind our house. It was a lovely day and the horses seemed eager to go, too.

It was the first time Boogie had been ridden outside of our field. I had *ponied* him and he would happily go anywhere with us. That day I wanted to ride him bareback, but you couldn't ride him bareback, so I put a saddle on him. I didn't like riding in a saddle, so it was harder for me than riding Clypso bareback. I was having a hard time staying on him for some reason. Clypso was safe. He could be a handful, but if you said, "Okay!" then he'd be nice. As the more inexperienced rider, Doug rode Clypso and I rode Boogie.

It was a bright, nearly cloudless day. There was a light breeze that made the tall, dry grass sway. The wind rattled the dry leaves that still clung to some of the trees. The noises made the horses a little more nervous—attentive, really—so we knew that we had to be a little bit more careful and aware of sights and sounds around us.

The horses were very alert and would snort nervously every so often. We rode by a lot of things that got their attention and we gently guided them along. The kids who lived on the land behind us had set up a paintball course in the woods that included an old bathtub and lots of other new things that we, and the horses, noticed along the way.

We rode further into the woods letting the horses adjust to the changes in the environment at their own pace. When we got all the way back into the woods, the neighbor kids drove up on their ATV. There was one ATV and a couple of kids on foot, so we stopped as they approached to keep the horses calm. The kids turned off the ATV and came up to talk with us for a little while. The horses saw them, accepted their presence, and relaxed.

We walked over to say hello and chat about the new paintball course. When we were ready to get going, we said goodbye.

It had crossed my mind, but we didn't ask them to wait to start the ATV until we had gotten farther away because the horses weren't spooked by the sound when they first approached us. Horses are prey animals in the wild. If they can see something and understand that it isn't a threat, they're usually fine. But noisy objects behind them can freak them out.

We turned and nudged our horses to walk on. When we were somewhere between fifty and a hundred feet away from the kids, they cranked up the ATV behind us.

Immediately, both our horses took off at a full gallop. It felt like warp five! We were not in control, and being deep in the woods was a bad place to not be in control.

Suddenly, we were rushing through brush and trees that were as high as we were, dodging bigger trees all around us. There was a trail, but we weren't headed for it.

Paula and I were separated by about fifteen feet as the horses ran away with us, with me on her left. I glimpsed over at her a couple of times as we sped along. I wasn't used to riding at a full gallop and she wasn't used to riding in a saddle; a frightening combination.

She was an accomplished rider, but for some reason, she just didn't stay on that day. Her right foot slipped out of the stirrup. I watched in horror as I saw her slide off Boogie and hit the ground, hard.

I've fallen off my share of horses and I never remember getting hurt badly from a fall. I remember always getting up after a fall, dusting myself off, and getting back on the horse. That's not what happened this time. The last thing I remember was starting to ride away after talking to those kids and our horses starting to run away, and nothing after that.

For some reason, I guess that my foot slipped out of the right stirrup and I fell off. I've heard that it's not the fall that hurts; it's the sudden stop at the end of it. I'm here to tell you that is absolutely true. This book is about what happened after that sudden stop as I hit the ground hard, and the lessons we can offer to those who have, or are yet to have, similar experiences.

I immediately pulled back hard on Clypso's reins. I pulled so hard that I got burns on a couple of my fingers. I turned him hard and when he stopped, I jumped off and let him go.

I ran to where Paula lay. When she hit the earth, she slid along the ground and came to rest in the root structure of an oak tree. Her neck was bent almost ninety degrees to the left—I was quite sure it was broken.

She wasn't wearing a helmet. Some people would say she was foolish, and I understand that. It's quite possible though, that the extra padding in the helmet might have snapped her neck, killing her instantly.

In any event, the force of her head hitting the ground was enough to cause terrible concussive forces with or without a helmet. We'll never know what difference it might have made now.

Luckily, the kids with the ATV were still nearby and saw what happened. I yelled, "Go home, call 911, and get an ambulance here right away!"

They took off on the ATV and I lost focus. Paula was out cold. I did the quick first aid review for bleeding, breathing, and shock. There didn't seem to be any bleeding or obviously broken bones. She was unconscious and breathing, but very shallowly. I considered whether it was better to move her or not to move her and decided against moving her.

Years of military discipline and training probably helped me a little, but I went into shock as well. I wasn't processing the situation as well as I might have. Time moved in very slow motion. I remember thinking that I needed to get the horses and dogs gathered up and back to the barn.

I asked one of the kids who were still with us to come over and stay with Paula while I went to find the horses. Our field was only a couple of hundred feet away from the site of the accident, so I figured I could go to the back gate and put the horses in the field and return pretty quickly.

It took a little bit longer for me to catch the horses than I anticipated, but I returned as soon as I could. I was at a loss as to what to do for Paula. None of my life experiences or training was serving either of us at this point. There was nothing apparent that I needed to do, or could do, other than take my vest off and put it gently over her to keep her warm.

The last thing that I remember is talking to those kids and leaving and the horses being spooked. I remember the horses starting to run away; and nothing after that.

It seemed like hours passed.

I have no sense of how long it really took until the paramedics arrived and began to do what they do best. They put Paula on a backboard, and it seemed to take a very long time to get her ready to go.

They said, "We've got to get her to the hospital." When I asked which hospital, they told me they were taking her to the Level I trauma unit at Akron City Hospital. I told them I would change my pants and meet them there.

I went home, changed clothes, put the dogs in the house, and took off for the hospital. I arrived about twenty-eight minutes later.

# Chapter 5

# What Do We Do Now?

I assumed that Paula was already there when I walked into the Akron City Hospital emergency room. I stepped up to the lady at the desk and said, "I'm Paula Poad's husband. Where is she?" When she replied, "We don't have a Paula Poad here," my blood ran cold. "What?!" I said. "The ambulance driver said they were bringing her here. Check again. Is she here?"

She checked again, but the hospital not only had no record of who she was or what was going on, they did not have Paula and were not responsible for knowing anything about her or her whereabouts.

The wonderful young lady at the reception desk called all the other hospitals in the area trying to help me find Paula. Finally, she hollered over to me, "I found her! She's in Ravenna and they are getting ready to put her on a helicopter. She'll be here in about an hour."

You've heard people say, "That was the longest hour of my life," without really appreciating what they meant, but this really was the longest hour of my life because I had no idea if Paula was dead or alive or somewhere still in between. My imagination ran wild with awful possibilities.

It turns out that the ambulance paramedics hadn't called Akron City Hospital to tell them they were taking Paula to Robinson Hospital in Portage County, a hospital halfway between our house and the one where I was waiting. It's a medium-sized facility in Ravenna with an emergency room but no Level I trauma center.

What made the ambulance stop at that hospital? I never did get, nor did I ever really push for, an answer. I did find out that at Robinson, they did some imaging and gave Paula Mannitol, a drug that helps reduce swelling in the brain.

It was another forty minutes before Paula's arrival at Akron City Hospital, not enough time for me to drive over to Robinson Hospital and accompany her on the flight, which I probably couldn't have done anyway.

While I waited, my thoughts cleared a bit and I went into mission mode, a single-minded focus on the problem at hand and what must be done to solve it. This is how I was trained to deal with situations during my navy career. I asked the woman at the reception desk what the plan was when Paula arrived.

She made some calls and told me that Dr. Markarian was the neurosurgeon on call. "Okay, is he here?" I asked. She replied, "He's just getting through with an emergency surgery, so he will be here and be available soon."

Then I called my boss, who was also a good friend, to tell

her what had happened. I wanted her to know about Paula and make arrangements for the classes that I was supposed to be teaching the following week. I called our neighbors to ask them to go over and let the dogs out in a couple of hours—taking care of the routines of our lives.

Still waiting, I walked out into the parking lot and saw a guy in a suit with a little wooden box. I don't know why I knew this but I suspected that in that box were the operating glasses that neurosurgeons use.

I walked up to the man and said, "Excuse me, are you Dr. Markarian?" and he replied, "Yes, why do you ask?"

I told him, "Well, you probably got a call that there is a lady coming in with either a broken neck or head injuries or something. That's my wife. I was riding with her when it happened. Let's talk about what's next."

We talked for a little bit, and instead of heading out to his car as he was doing, he turned around to walk in with me. We got a chance to talk for a little longer.

Soon my neighbor drove up and was with me when the helicopter came. That's something that I don't wish on anybody, watching a loved one come out of the back end of a helicopter. Something in you expects them to be alert so you can run over, hug them, and say "Hi!" But you can't do any of that. The area under and around the helicopter is off-limits for safety reasons.

When they take your loved one out, they rush him or her into the emergency room because, after all, it is an emergency if they are flying to the hospital in a helicopter. All I could do was stand about a hundred feet away, watch her being moved, and wish it weren't happening.

I first saw Paula again in the trauma room. She was alive but still unconscious. The nurse had taken Paula's jewelry off and cut away her clothes. She put her jewelry in a bag and handed it to me. I stuffed it in my pocket, trying not to think that she may never wear it again.

I was in the way while they worked on her, but I really didn't want to leave. I imagined that this might well be the last time I was ever going to see her alive.

There is something in that moment when you take the personal items in your hand that belong to your loved one—your best friend, your spouse—that instantly changes you. It may be a kind of pre-grieving thing; like a goodbye that you don't want to happen.

If Paula had broken a leg, I'd take her jewelry home and I would know that it would be there when she got home. But in that moment, it seemed like I was taking her jewelry knowing that she might not be coming back home and might never wear it again.

Based on what I'd heard up to this point, I thought there was greater than a fifty percent chance that she would die. I remember whispering in her ear as she lay on that emergency room gurney, "I love you; thanks for everything we've had together. I hope you get through this so we can fight on the other side." This was so different, and harder, than anything I'd ever done before that I can hardly describe it or the emotions that were flooding my brain.

They did a computerized tomography (CT) scan and other triage activities, and in twenty minutes or so the neurosurgeon took me into one of those little consult rooms.

He had the CT scan in front of him and said, "This doesn't look good. She is really in pretty bad shape."

Still in mission mode, I said, "I know. How bad is it and what can we do?"

He showed me the scan and almost the entire brain cavity was white. The neurosurgeon explained to me, "This is supposed to be all dark, but it's all white which means her skull is full of blood. That's not good because blood is toxic to brain cells."

He told me, "There's probably only a fifty-fifty chance that she will survive."

I very clearly remember replying, "So why are we sitting here talking? We're burning daylight! Get in there and fix her!"

Some might view my reaction as cold and detached, but falling apart and panicking wouldn't have helped Paula. Helping her survive and recover was my primary mission in life at that point.

Dr. Markarian left me and met Paula in the operating room. I went to a waiting area that felt like a movie theater lobby after closing time; cold, empty, and alone. I was full of anxiety, fear, and any other negative emotion you can think of while Paula was in surgery.

Every time a door opened, I looked to see if it was the doctor. I wanted to know something; anything. Time stood nearly still. I was hugely relieved when Dr. Markarian came out about four-and-a-half, long hours later and told me, "Well, she survived surgery. She's getting cleaned up and will be on her way up to recovery for a little while. You can't go in and see her yet, but they will let you know when she is up in ICU."

# CHAPTER 6

# WAITING IS...
# LEARNING WHAT SURVIVAL
# IS ALL ABOUT

While I was waiting to hear the results of Paula's surgery, three people arrived to be with me: my boss, her husband, and another neighbor. They hugged me and offered some words of encouragement, condolence, or comfort that I frankly didn't hear, but their presence was a great comfort.

I found that I was excusing myself a lot to walk around the hospital; I needed the alone time. I'd call family and other friends to update them on any new developments. I wasn't as interested in providing them with updates as I was in hearing the voices of people I cared for and who cared for us.

Sometimes I'd find an isolated quiet spot and scream a little bit. I'd get a cup of coffee. Having people present for me gave me a new sensitivity. Prior to the accident, I wouldn't have been one of those guys who would go out walking with somebody who needed support. But now, I am that kind of guy that says, "What can I do to help? Whatever it is, let me know and I'll either sit here with you or go away."

Sometimes I felt like I didn't have the energy to be comforted. But I knew that people were there for me, and I came back and talked to them occasionally.

At the time, I worked at Mount Union College, a truly awesome place. We had about 1,900 students, but it felt to me like a very close-knit family. When she showed up in the ER, my boss hugged me and told me, "I talked to the president and we've got your back. He said to tell you to go do what you need to do and come back as soon as you can. We've also got your classes covered."

The college and the people there were just amazingly supportive. I didn't have to take a leave of absence. When Paula went to the rehabilitation hospital for five months, my boss drove the three miles over to our house every morning and evening to feed and water the horses and muck the stalls when I couldn't be home. She had thirty horses of her own, but still came over to take care of our two horses, two dogs, and two cats.

Later, we learned that Dr. Markarian was younger than many of the other neurosurgeons we met, which also meant that he didn't have the years of experience that older doctors did. That didn't mean that he was unskilled, though. I'm convinced that he was able to help Paula survive because he was younger and full of the most current knowledge. He is an exceptionally talented neurosurgeon and an amazing man.

Between the time Dr. Markarian talked to me and the first

time I saw her after surgery in the ICU, I had gained a great deal of confidence in him.

When I walked into Paula's ICU room around 11:30 that night, they had cleaned her up so she was all fresh-faced, pink, and scrubbed. But she also had tubes and wires of all sorts, including what looked like a car's spark plug screwed into the top of her head.

I was tremendously naive. I distinctly remember walking into her ICU room, seeing her all hooked up, and thinking to myself, "Man, this sucks. Look at all these tubes. She's going to be in here for at least three or four days."

I soon learned just how laughable that thought was. There are no words I have found to adequately describe how ignorant I was about how our lives had just changed and what it was going to take to work through it all.

The spark plug, for instance, was called an intracranial pressure monitor. With head injuries, one of the problems is that the patient's cranial pressure can build up so much that it can actually force the brain down through the bottom of the skull.

That night in surgery, Dr. Markarian did a procedure called a craniotomy. He removed a part of her skull, bigger than my hand, on the left side of her head from a point just behind her left eye, back across the top of her ear, around to the back of her head, and back up almost through the center of her head on top to the front. He did this to relieve pressure from the swelling and buildup of fluids that happens when the brain is injured.

This was a pretty astounding thing to hear about, but Dr. Markarian told me that if they had not done it, the pressure buildup would have given her brain no way to swell and heal, and she would likely have died.

This was the first of many times that I appreciated Dr. Markarian's energy, skills, and genuine compassion.

The next several days were full of new things to learn on the journey of survival with many procedures, tests, and other things I had never heard of.

I was experiencing something akin to bunker mentality, an army term used to describe being in a bunker in the middle of a battle with shells falling all around you and bullets whizzing by. You feel like you're standing on the interstate and cars are zooming by. You're walking in the same direction as the cars are moving, but you're not getting anywhere, just trying to stay aware and alive.

Bunker mentality is a state of shock. Things are moving very fast and you feel like you have no control, most often because you don't. You are present, but not really aware or able to function normally. You keep your head down until the shelling stops.

Things were going on that I didn't understand. All the monitors, for instance. I was learning what they were measuring, because I wanted to know what that little spark plug did, but I really couldn't do anything to affect the decisions being made on her behalf to keep her alive. It all changed so quickly in response to her constantly changing condition.

Paula was in what is technically called a coma, or extended recovery. I later found out she was going to be in a coma for a couple of weeks at least.

It's like cats when they feel bad, they go lie down and don't wake up until they're okay. I did what a cat does; I went and lay down to heal.

My understanding of the word coma had come mostly from TV shows where somebody is asleep, then they suddenly open their eyes and start talking about the dog or what they wanted for breakfast, and poof, they're fully awake.

That's not the way it happens in real life, because the transition from being in a coma to being awake took many days. Paula would move a little now and then, but we didn't really know if she was awake, or in a coma, or what was going on.

While she was in the ICU, I really struggled, wondering if she was in what I traditionally thought of as a coma and thinking that if she just "came out of it," things would be all right.

I looked for milestones. Coming out of a coma was a milestone that I could check off my mental list and think, "Progress!" But I learned that it's not one check box, it's a series of check boxes.

Up to this point, I had already learned many things that no one should have to learn about surviving and recovering from traumatic brain injury. But they must be learned if we are going to help our loved ones survive.

About halfway through Paula's time in the ICU, I got a book from the hospital, *Living with Brain Injury* written by a doctor from HealthSouth, which helped me learn a lot of the technical stuff.

I started researching with intensity. I looked at information, questions, and answers in books on head injuries. I kept track of what I found and if I had questions, I would write them down and ask the doctor whenever I saw him.

The hospital staff thought I was pretty weird because I was more inquisitive and not in as much shock anymore. They observed me in mission mode. This was my way of getting organized to help Paula fight and survive.

My mind wandered, sometimes productively and sometimes destructively. I fought hard not to let it wander into dark corners full of fear and self-pity.

About three days into this whole ordeal, it occurred to me that part of my job at Mount Union was to supervise interns and help them process new and challenging situations. I would ask them to capture their activities and thoughts in a daily journal, then reflect on them and learn from their own writings. So I said to myself, "Get yourself a notebook and journal to help you collect your thoughts. It'll help you deal with this whole thing, even if nobody ever reads it."

After lunch, I walked over to the drugstore and bought a notebook. I started writing by backfilling what had happened over the first three days and bringing my/our experiences to the current moment.

The journal starts on February 9. Seventy-nine pages later on July 14, I decided that I either couldn't continue writing, or didn't need to.

# CHAPTER 7

# WHEN WEEKS
# FEEL LIKE MONTHS

When I got home after seeing Paula in the ICU that first night, I drafted a brief email to a large group of our family, friends, and acquaintances with a recount of exactly what was going on and where we were.

I wrote, "When I left, she was in ICU," which started a long two-way conversation with all those folks. I received countless reassuring responses and I felt part of an extended network of support and care.

Coming home without Paula that first night was awful. I was tired, so I cranked up the tunes and cried on the way home. Then I cried some more at home. But I couldn't just sit around and cry, so I went and sent that email.

The bed was too big that night and the dogs got a lot closer to me because I hugged them for comfort. It was so surreal because I didn't know if she was ever going to be on the other side of the bed again. I knew it was a possibility and I started trying to come to grips with the idea of being alone. I missed Paula like no other time in my life. It scared me a lot.

When I asked the hospital when the next ICU visiting hours were, they told me to come at 8:00 in the morning and I would get thirty minutes to see her. I found this out at 11:30 p.m. I slept hard for about three hours; I was exhausted. I didn't feel anything like normal.

I set the alarm for 4:30 a.m. so I could get up, take a shower and shave, feed the horses, put the dogs out in the barn because they couldn't be in the house, and get my butt to the hospital to see her as quickly as I could.

At the hospital, I had a long talk with the doctor and asked what the milestones were that would tell us if she was going to make it. I asked when we might know whether Paula was going to survive. He said, "The next forty-eight hours are critical. If she survives the next forty-eight, it's a really good sign. But it's not a determining sign. You'll have a lot of work ahead of you and so will she."

Then he told me something that he knew to be true, but was probably the scariest thing I had heard up until then. "This head injury is one of the more severe I have seen and there is no reason that she should survive it. Her whole skull was full of blood."

We found out later that Paula had a half-inch hole in one of the two main veins that return the blood from the brain to the heart, and it was leaking blood into the inside her skull where it really didn't belong. They removed a piece of her left temporal lobe the size of a ping pong ball because the internal bleeding had killed it.

When your head hits the ground like that, with or without a helmet, it's a severe concussion because your head stops moving, but your brain doesn't. It slams around inside the skull causing tremendous damage. The brain's connections get stretched, ripped apart, and some of them die. The same goes for the actual brain itself. All that internal impact does damage, and some of it doesn't recover.

We're not crash test dummies. Dr. Markarian broke it down for me. "Consider this analogy: Think about what would happen if all the phone lines in the entire world were blown down all at once and have to be restrung. Some of them aren't going to get rewired properly, and it is going to take a very long time to get the job done."

That conversation became the model for our recovery.

I also use the analogy of reformatting your hard drive and reloading all the programs one at a time, and then going in to change all the configurations and get them working again by testing each of them. Each of these programs is like a different system in your body: sight, taste, muscle control, and everything you are and do. After an accident like Paula's, every program has to be reinstalled. In the telephone line analogy, the problem is that it is being done by electricians who are each working at their own pace. They take breaks; they go on vacation, they make mistakes, and sometimes get things wrong.

The ICU waiting room is an interesting ecosystem. When I was there, there were anywhere from five to twelve patients in the ICU and the visiting hours were very short, only a half hour, twice a day. One at 8:00 a.m. and one at 2:00 p.m. Occasionally they'd let you in once at night.

After three days, I pretty much ignored the rules and went in whenever the heck I wanted to. The staff was okay with that. I told them, "I don't want to be in the waiting room if there's a possibility that I would miss my last chance to see her alive. If she's going to go, I want to be there. I could be in there stroking her arm, touching her."

One thing I am quite sure of is that people in a coma are present, even if they can't communicate. I made sure that I was as positive and upbeat as possible when I was in her room, even if I wasn't feeling it. I didn't want any negativity in the room so I made sure that anyone else that went in there was also positive and upbeat.

I would go in to her room and tell her how the horses and the dogs were to help keep her in the present moment. I'd tell her that they were doing fine and looking forward to seeing her.

I would stroke and hold Paula's hands and ask, "Can you squeeze?" It was an ongoing neurological test, but really, I was just being there with her and connecting in any way that I could. Surprisingly, she could squeeze my hand a lot earlier than she could do anything else. I wondered if that meant she was still in a coma.

It didn't matter. What mattered was that she squeezed my hand. She wasn't talking yet. She didn't open her eyes. She wasn't alert, so technically they wouldn't say she was out of a coma. But I'd think about how she just squeezed my hand, so how can she be in a coma? That definition is still fuzzy and that word really didn't hold any meaning to me anymore.

The ICU waiting room was like a tide coming in and out. The families would go in and visit their loved one and then come back out and you could see what the news was by how the families acted when they came out.

I remember people whose loved ones died. After two days or more of seeing the same people, I'd go over and we'd hug when they came back into the waiting room. We were sharing things that made us seem almost like a family. We were a *community of waiters* held together by these common bonds of fear, uncertainty, and hope. We shared one another's stories.

Personally, I found that those relationships and those brief moments of support were even more valuable than the support of even my family and friends who didn't—and couldn't possibly—understand what I was experiencing.

After two days, the doctors provided new milestones, and it became clear that she was more than likely going to survive. I didn't know what the next steps were yet, but the promise of survival was uplifting.

It seemed to me that a lot of the folks in an ICU waiting room don't go home happy because their loved ones die. That not only takes a toll on the families, but on the nurses and doctors who work there. The staff is amazing to me. I really don't think they just look at a patient coming in and say, "Oh, there's another one. Chalk one up for the bad side." I think they struggle when someone doesn't recover. I know they seemed to fight hard for Paula and me.

Paula was mostly bald. They weren't really careful about shaving the hair on the right side, and the left side was completely bald. But she looked better than Kirstie Alley in Star Trek. She pulled off bald very well.

I don't do bald good.

I expected to see a lot of damage there because the doctor

had said, "We took out a piece of her skull. It's in the freezer here." I expected to see something very different, but the left side of her head where they took out the piece of skull was perfectly round and looked like it was intact. They didn't have a big dressing on it; just sutures because they left it open to allow the brain to swell and shrink and heal on its own time.

Paula had several things develop that required actions I really didn't understand at the time. There were procedures that I had never heard about and lots of tests, imaging, and blood work. I had to learn what was going on so I could get a feel for where we were and what was happening.

One time, Paula had blood clots in her right leg because she wasn't moving it. Blood clots in your leg are not good because they can travel to your brain, your heart, your lungs, and can kill you.

The doctor started her on blood thinners. I guess they worked a little too well, because she started having blood in her urine. They said, "That's not doing what we really wanted it to do, so let's go to plan B." They decided that they were going to insert what is called a Greenfield filter.

The doctor came to me and said, "We are going to insert a Greenfield filter. Don't worry, this is routine."

This sort of set me off. I told him, "Two things you need to hear. First, I don't know what a Greenfield filter is. And second, you need to quit using that word 'routine,' because none of this is routine for me. It might be routine for you and I really do appreciate that; I'm glad it's routine because that means that you've done it before and that you're probably pretty good at it. Know that if I hear you saying this is pretty extraordinary, I'm going to get real nervous."

The doctor explained to me that a Greenfield filter is a little titanium umbrella that they insert in her inferior vena cava, the main vein that returns blood from the lower body. It's a little umbrella that opens up inside the vein, catches blood clots, and lets them dissolve.

"Oh, okay. It still doesn't sound routine to me, but I'll approve it," I told him. I had to sign all the medical disclaimers and approvals. Then they scheduled more routine treatment protocols, like a tracheotomy, because she couldn't breathe for herself after surgery. Maybe she could breathe on her own and maybe she couldn't, but they couldn't trust her body to do it on its own.

They also inserted a feeding tube into her stomach into which they pumped some sort of brownish food mixture. It looked to me as though someone had already eaten it, but they assured me that it was really good for her and had everything she needed in it. I never asked to taste it, though.

I wondered if my desire to have us moving forward, knowing what we were doing and how it was helping her recover was a good thing or a bad thing. Putting in a feeding tube sounded to me like it was a step backward, but I found out that it was a good thing because it meant that she could process food. We could trust her digestive system, whereas we couldn't two days beforehand. I started to see that something that might look horrible and invasive was probably a good thing. This helped me appreciate that with a severe head injury, all the body's systems have to come back on and be tested before they can be relied upon to continue working correctly.

One of the things that the doctor told me was, "You know, you've got a long recovery here." I asked, "How long?" He said, "Well, I can't tell you because every head injury is different.

If you've met one person with a head injury, then you've met one person with a head injury. Everyone is different and there is no playbook. There are protocols. If this happens, we do that..."

They have a general plan of what they know they need to do and what they are watching for. I got up to speed on a lot of those possible outcomes so I could relate it to myself and plan accordingly, but there were a lot of speed bumps.

Many doctors told me that we were going to have days where you take one or two steps forward. You're also going to have days where you take one step back or maybe even two or three steps back. But as long as you're taking more steps forward than you've taken back over time, you're making progress. That's just how you have to judge things. I told them I could deal with that. "When something happens, don't tell me it's routine. Tell me this is a step forward or a step back. I may not know, and I need to know," I explained to them.

We also saw things like the time in the hospital in Pittsburgh when Paula was having her bone flap (skull pieces) put back in. When the nurse came in and changed her IV bag and started the pump, she didn't hook the tube up to her arm. The machine was pumping all her meds and IV fluids out on the floor for about five minutes. I heard something dripping, checked it out, and told the nurse, "I'm pretty sure that's not right." The nurse had been tired and preoccupied.

Mistakes often happen not because they are bad nurses or uncaring people; they were almost always phenomenally caring and capable people doing the best they could under the circumstances.

Overall, the staff at the hospital in Akron was awesome. We went back later, after Paula could talk a little more, to say thank you. We took Paula back to the emergency room. We found the same woman that helped me find out where she was that first day when she was missing. By that point, Paula was using a walker and we walked in together. I said, "This is the lady that you helped me find six months ago. Thank you."

We all had a hug and shared some goose bumps and a few tears, but this time they were tears of joy and gratitude. We also went up to the ICU and visited a bit with the nurses and staff on duty at that time. One of the reasons I brought Paula back afterwards is because they have such amazing attitudes toward patients.

I also wanted them to see one of the happy endings that they were a part of so that they can visualize more of them when they are working with future patients.

I felt comfortable not being there with Paula for some of the time in the ICU because of the quality of the staff, but one thing I learned is, if you have a loved one in the hospital, you need to be there to advocate on their behalf. Somebody needs to be with them to watch for things that don't make sense and to ask the hard questions about what's going on and what needs to be done.

One morning, I came in to her ICU room and there was a box of chocolates, a bottle of wine, and a note from one of Paula's friends from New Jersey. She had been hauling some horses to Youngstown, Ohio and came the extra forty miles or so to see Paula very early in the morning. Paula may not have known that she came by, but I'm of the mind that she did.

I brought donuts to the ICU nurses and tried to be both friendly and appreciative of their efforts, which was helpful because they looked the other way when we sort of snuck the therapy dog in to see Paula. I'm not exactly sure whether I actually snuck the dog in, but I sure didn't ask permission. The therapy dog handler didn't object. I said, "Come on, we're going to the ICU. My wife is in there and she loves dogs."

This was about two-and-a-half weeks after the accident. It was a large black dog with long hair, and he sat down beside Paula's bed. I placed her left hand on the dog's head. She started scratching instinctively. She still wasn't clearly awake and alert; she hadn't even opened her eyes yet, but she was petting the dog. There was no doubt in my mind that she knew she was petting a dog again, though, and that she was enjoying it.

I did a lot of things in the ICU to try to communicate with her. I talked to her. I brought a CD player and played some of her favorite music from time to time. I knew that she could sense something outside of herself in her environment. I couldn't deal with her not being there. I warned people who came to see her while she was *sleeping* that we needed to assume that she could hear everything we were saying, and not to say anything negative while in the room with her.

I watched a lot of moments where people were showing care and compassion to other people in the ICU. I saw what other people were going through and I had a lot of spare time on my hands. It made me feel better to recognize them and say, "Thank you. I know what you're going through by watching you."

I spent a lot of time walking around thinking. It was a big hospital and I got to know a lot of the corridors and nooks and crannies while I was walking and thinking. One of the things I realized I needed to do was identify my mission objectives. I went back to my military mode of asking questions: What do we have to accomplish to get her better? What can I do to help?

I also went through the pre-grieving process, if you will. Grief incorporates shock, anger, denial, and finally acceptance. I went through all those emotions. Was I in denial when I looked at Paula and said, "She's going to be in here for three or four days?" Probably. But when I reached acceptance, I said, "Okay. Now what do we need to do?"

Later, I started bringing her jewelry back.

One day, I leaned down and kissed her on the lips and she kissed back. That was stellar! That made my whole day. I knew that Paula would have to do a lot of work and I knew the doctors were important, but I wondered what I should be doing to help. I wanted to figure out our next step–when, not if, but when she gets out of the ICU, where do we want to go? The social workers, doctors, and I started talking about when and how to move her to a rehab hospital and how to pick a good one.

Through my research online, reading *Living With Brain Injury*, and talking to the doctors and social workers, I learned that the faster you get somebody with a brain injury (an injury or a stroke, because they are both brain injuries) into rehab, the better their recovery is going to be. You could say that you're prodding those electricians to work faster.

After she was clearer, not out of her coma, but at least in what they called the clearing stage, I started to get pretty pushy about getting her into rehab as soon as possible. I asked the ICU staff when we could transfer her and started looking at options.

At first I researched the locations of the best rehab hospitals in the country. I didn't want to go to the local rehab facility just because it happened to be in my hometown. If we had to travel far away to get her in a good one, then we would do it and figure out how to make it work later.

I identified three top rehab hospitals in the country: One in Colorado, one in Texas (both of which I understand that Gabby Giffords, the senator from Arizona who was shot by a would-be assassin, was in at one time or another), and a third one called HealthSouth in Monroeville, Pennsylvania, about an hour and a half east of where we lived. Ironically, this one was about eight miles away from my sister's house. I said to myself, "This will work!" I drove there and met with the people at HealthSouth toward the end of Paula's time in the ICU.

After discussing Paula's case and what was going on, they said, "We could take her tomorrow in her current condition." The facility is part of a nationwide chain and was very highly regarded. They had a dedicated wing for patients with head injuries and could even take people in on full respiratory support, in other words, on a respirator.

After I saw what they could offer, my mission shifted to getting Paula admitted to their facility as soon as possible.

When I look back on our situation, I realize that I was in one of the best possible positions to deal with this catastrophe; probably better off than ninety-eight percent of the people that have to work through such an ordeal. I wasn't going to lose my job if I went to the hospital too much. I had good medical insurance from the navy retirement. I had my retired navy pay. Money, time, and my ability to focus on what needed to be done were not going to be hindrances in my helping Paula to heal and recover. I had supportive family who happened to live close to one of my facilities of choice.

These were huge, positive factors in our ability to do what we needed to do. I cannot begin to do an adequate job of expressing my gratitude to the people who were there to support us as Paula fought to survive. My sister and her husband were the absolute embodiment of loving support. I'm not sure I could have made it through this without their support. I'm tremendously sensitive to the idea that not everybody would be able or willing to do what I did. Our friend, Aik Teong, was also a great source of support and comfort to both of us and remains so to this day.

Other people might have to work a forty-hour week while their loved one was in the hospital. I don't know how to make up for that, but I recognize that I'm enormously blessed to be in a position to be as present as I was in the survival phase.

Toward the end of her stay in the ICU, Paula was getting better and it became clear that she was going to survive. Fewer crises developed and the doctors were less guarded with their comments; they no longer couched their comments in nuanced language because her survival became more of a certainty.

We now needed to think about driving her recovery, and that included moving her from the hospital to HealthSouth as soon as possible. I was not aggressive enough in coordinating Paula's move to Monroeville with my health insurance company early enough, though. I became a nuisance to the hospital as I didn't know that we needed pre-authorizations from my insurance company, or how that all worked. I just figured we would get her in an ambulance, get on the road to Monroeville, and take care of the paperwork later. I just sort of told them we wanted to get her to HealthSouth and pushed them to make it happen ASAP. I counted on the social workers at the hospital to start the process, but I soon learned that it takes longer than I gave them. After some backtracking and cajoling, it worked out.

I wanted to move Paula to HealthSouth directly from ICU, and they were ready for her to come. I had done all the paperwork to get her in there. I didn't know that the insurance company wasn't moving as fast as we needed in order to get her into an ambulance to transfer her. The hospital was also uncomfortable releasing her until she had been on a medical/surgical floor for a couple of days. They wanted to follow protocol, especially with Paula still on a respirator.

But I was against that because the hospital knew the quality of HealthSouth, that their dedicated head trauma unit was one of the best, and that I wanted Paula there as quickly as possible to improve her recovery. That was a little problem at the end that we had to work through. It took five or six days longer than I wanted, but it happened, and the ambulance showed up at the hospital one day to take her to Monroeville for the long drive to recovery that lay ahead.

# PART TWO:

# DRIVE

Drive (drahyv) - An innate, biologically determined urge to attain a goal or satisfy a need.

*"Let us not be content to wait and see what will happen, but give us the determination to make the right things happen."*
—Horace Mann

Part Two is all about working hard, working together, and driving to recover as much of Paula's former self as we possibly can. I say *can* and not *could* because this is an ongoing effort. Paula continues to work hard and make improvements and I continue to work hard to help her do so. We have every expectation that she will continue to recover far into our future together.

Friedrich Nietzsche is credited with having said, "That which does not kill us makes us stronger." That is not necessarily true. Don't get me wrong, survival is great, but getting stronger after a traumatic brain injury is hard work and takes an entirely different focus and motivation than just surviving.

Survival, in Paula's case, depended mostly on the knowledge and work of others. Sure, her naturally positive attitude played a major part, but the skill, dedication, and hard work of the first responders, her doctors, nurses, me, family members, and friends had a more direct, tangible impact in those early days.

Part Two is also about celebrating the work of the next group of professionals, the therapists who drove her to work hard and helped her move from one goal to the next. More importantly, this section is about Paula's stubbornness and desire to please others by getting better and recovering as much of her former self as she could. To a lesser extent, it is also about the roles that I and other family members and friends played. In the final analysis, it is about hard work, hope, love, and healing from traumatic brain injury, which is the subtitle of this book and the most important stage once you've survived the initial trauma.

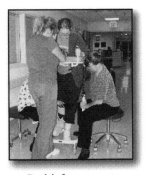

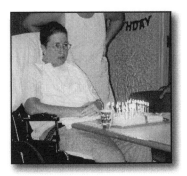

Paula's first steps at HealthSouth. Many caring hands make magic happen

Paula's 46th birthday party at HealthSouth - 5 months after her injury

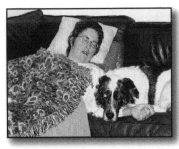

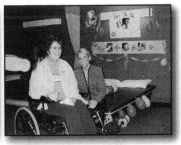

Paula's first day back home - on the couch relaxing with one of our furry kids

Celebrating a year of progress in physical therapy with her therapy team

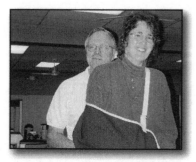

Paula on the treadmill at
physical therapy with Doug spotting
her from behind

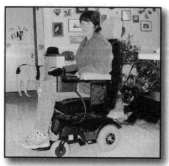

Paula's indoor mobility that
helped her get around and do
more things on her own

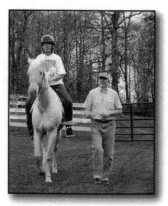

Paula back in the saddle again,
therapeutic riding
at Pegasus Farm

# CHAPTER 8

# DRIVING TO RECOVER

Paula was in the hospital for almost four weeks before she was finally moved to HealthSouth, with all but a couple of those days being spent in the ICU.

It was early March of 2002 when they loaded her into the ambulance and headed for Monroeville. Aik Teong, a friend of ours, and I followed the ambulance for the whole two-hour drive from Akron City Hospital to HealthSouth. We jumped out of our car and were waiting when they opened the ambulance door and got Paula out.

Although Paula was awake, smiling and waving at us when she was taken upstairs from the ambulance, she has said that the first thing she remembers is waking up in a private room about two days after she arrived.

When she went into the ambulance, I told her I'd meet her in Monroeville and she responded. She doesn't remember that exchange. Her body must have been totally focused inwardly on healing even if the outward expressions appeared normal and hopeful.

Aik Teong has played an important role in this story, too. We never had kids because we never really wanted them and our time in the navy was more enjoyable without them. We always had four-legged furry kids.

While I was teaching at Mount Union College, Paula and I became friends with Aik Teong, a young man from Malaysia, through an International Friends program that the college offered. He graduated three months after Paula had her accident. I still don't pronounce his name properly, but he is as much a part of our family as anyone related by blood.

When we refer to him as "The son we never knew we wanted," people look at us funny. What we mean is that we think of him as our son even though we never wanted to have children.

Before her accident, Paula and Aik Teong would take our dogs up to Cuyahoga Valley National Park and walk through the woods while I worked. They all loved that time together. He'd come out to our house for occasional weekends, Thanksgiving, and other school breaks. Sometimes he'd bring friends from school.

After graduating from Mount Union, he earned a Ph.D. and worked in a post-doctorate fellowship researching cancer at the UCLA Medical Center. He would send us papers he authored or coauthored that were published during his graduate studies and post-doctorate fellowship and I'd ask him, "Can you send one with more pictures? And I'm not talking about pictures of organic chemistry chains."

He's smart as a whip. He leaned down to talk to me and I'd think, "Thank you so much."

She's right; he's one of the smartest people I know.

When Paula had her accident and was in the hospital in Akron, Aik Teong was still a senior in college. He had limited opportunities to go to the hospital; he couldn't skip school to come and spend a day. He would get a ride up with a friend or I'd pick him up and we'd stop for dinner and go to the hospital at night once or twice a week so that he could spend some time with Paula.

Her injury affected him deeply, too. We'd had a close relationship with him for a year and a half before the accident. We still talk once or twice a week, but don't see him enough because he's in California and we're in North Carolina.

I stayed in Monroeville the whole first week Paula was at HealthSouth. After that, I stayed at my sister's house from Sunday through Thursday and went back to Ohio on Thursday afternoons. I'd spend time in my office at Mount Union on Friday, do some house and yard work on Saturday, and go back to Monroeville on Sunday morning.

When he graduated in May, Aik Teong stayed with me full time until he left to start his graduate school studies. He joined in the Ohio-Pennsylvania treks and stayed at my sister's house, too. He spent time with Paula at HealthSouth and would read her favorite stories to her. He helped me load hay for the horses in Ohio, build a ramp and sidewalk that Paula would need, and even helped me install the stair lift that she would need to get up and down the stairs to the second floor bedroom. His presence was important to both Paula and me. I think it was good for him to observe Paula's progress and appreciate how hard she worked to recover.

# CHAPTER 9

# SETTLING INTO HEALTHSOUTH FOR THE LONG DRIVE BACK

Paula got settled into her room at HealthSouth while I completed the check-in paperwork. The staff there was extremely professional.

HealthSouth had a main center section with a variety of wings, each dedicated to a different type of rehabilitation need. Clearly, the one I am most familiar with was the head trauma wing to treat traumatic brain injuries and acquired brain injuries such as strokes. The head trauma wing had specially trained nurses, dedicated physical therapists and occupational therapists that work with head injury patients as a primary role. They even had a recreational therapist whose job it was to provide therapeutically relevant activities and games for patients. I can't recommend the folks at HealthSouth highly enough.

I remember coming up from Never-Never Land when I was in the place in Monroeville. I remember a room with desks. I would be awake for about a half an hour and go to sleep and wake up and go to sleep and wake up. I don't remember what the therapists or doctors did. I do remember they'd come in and talk to me and I was in a pretty room and no one was there except for the people coming in and out. They washed my hair and cleaned me up and I had to stay in the room. I couldn't get around quite yet.

Someone on staff said that's when she actually came out of her coma. It certainly was a very clear line of demarcation; she was awake and alert and remembers.

The first night she was there, they freaked me out because they gave her a shower. She was breathing through a tracheotomy tube and had a feeding tube. I wondered how a shower was going to work. They told me, are you ready for this, not to worry, this is routine.

For the first time in over a month, I started to relax a bit when I heard that word. They got her in a big rolling chair, wheeled her into the shower, gave her a full-body shower, and washed her hair. In ICU, she had only received sponge baths. She didn't have much hair, so washing it was simpler in the hospital.

I bought her one of those turban style hats that people wear when they are doing chemotherapy, but she was pretty adamant that she wasn't going to be wearing it, so I donated it to a cancer wing at the nearby hospital.

I don't remember my sister visiting me in the ICU. I remember Doug saying that my sister was freaking out when she first saw me. My sister came to see me near the end of the time I was in the hospital in Akron. She was living in New Mexico and it was hard for her to get there. I don't remember much of anything from those days, though.

I remember being in the room and Aik Teong coming in and sitting and talking to me. Doug came and went more as he visited with me and dealt with the money, schedule, and other stuff. He was also working with his interns at Mount Union by email.

I have no memories of waking up and saying, "Wow. This happened. Bummer, dude." My brain will remember some of my past, though I can't remember the time early in the hospital. I remember being in the rehab room. I remember the people coming and going. I remember that I didn't do much therapy unless someone took me out of the room.

They were doing some therapy with her in the room, but not much. She was feeling things, and she still had a tracheotomy tube in her throat. She was breathing on her own, but it was through that tube in her throat. This actually kept her from being able to talk, since the air she was breathing wasn't going through her voice box. There was a device they put on the tracheotomy tube that allowed her to talk some, but it was very hard work. She wasn't very good at it, but got better with the help of her speech therapist. As she continued to improve, they worked on getting her to the point that they could remove that tracheotomy tube. When they finally did remove it, we saved it and burned it in a little ceremony back in one of our fields after she came home to Ohio.

She also had a feeding tube in her stomach when she got to HealthSouth—another one of those routine procedures that blew my mind. She was not able to eat anything because her mouth, throat, and brain weren't all reconnected and working right yet.

The nurses at Akron and later at HealthSouth mixed up some light brown liquid that resembled whole wheat pancake batter and let it flow into the tube that went from the outside of her body into her stomach. Getting rid of this tube was another one of those big milestones in the drive to recover, but she would need to be able to eat on her own first.

When the staff at HealthSouth determined that she should be able to handle eating food by mouth, they left the feeding tube in for a time and started her on something called a mechanical soft diet. The diet includes "foods that have a smoother consistency than regular foods. They require very little or no chewing at all to swallow." That doesn't do the diet justice.

She graduated from what resembled whole wheat pancake batter to what looked like baby food of various colors. They took whole food and blended it until it was a thicker liquid and easier to swallow. They even added something to thicken it more, since they were worried about it going down into her lungs if it weren't thicker.

It was amazing to watch her actually relearn how to swallow food under the watchful eye of her speech therapist. This part of her therapy was one of the things I had the most trouble understanding. I figured that we would just give Paula some food and see if she could eat it. It took several explanations, but I finally understood that we wouldn't know if a particular whole food was safe and that there was a significant chance that she might choke.

She was on the mechanical soft diet for about a month and a half. She actually took herself off it by eating the chocolate bow tie off a Vermont Teddy Bear that my nephew sent her, but more on that later.

They gave me this icky food. Then they moved me to another room and I would watch people. I would talk to anyone that was there. I remember one lady who was my first roommate in Monroeville, but she was never there, she was just off in La La land. I don't like private rooms. I like company.

Initially, Paula was in a private room at HealthSouth because they found Methicillin-resistant Staphylococcus aureus (MRSA) colonies in her nose and sinuses. According to The Mayo Clinic, staph bacteria are normally found on the skin or in the nose of about one-third of the population. The bacteria are generally harmless unless they enter the body through a cut or other wound, and even then they usually cause only minor skin problems in healthy people. But when those nasty little bugs get into a person's bloodstream, they wreak havoc and are often life-threatening, so her infection received immediate, aggressive attention at HealthSouth. This wasn't as much of a problem during the survival phase in Akron, as there were many more pressing things going on.

At HealthSouth, Paula was kept in an isolation room until she was rid of this MRSA infection. When she woke up there, she didn't like having the private room that came along with being in isolation. After a week or two, they determined that she didn't have and wasn't at risk of an actual MRSA infection, so they moved her to a regular room with her first roommate.

Paula had three or four roommates during her time there. One of the things I liked about HealthSouth is they didn't have private rooms; they had semi-private rooms and they were very deliberate about who they put in with you. Private rooms aren't good for recovery. Paula had an older roommate who had suffered a stroke, and then she had a middle-aged roommate. Her last roommate was a lady her age that had also fallen off a horse. This was a match made in heaven and they remain good friends even now.

Her family would come and I'd say hello and talk to them. At mealtimes, the staff had me in the cafeteria, sometimes a whole bunch of us would all be in a dining room. All these people who eat the weird soft food would be in a room, all sitting down. I don't know if we talked much. We just ate. I don't remember talking.

During lunchtime, they had a big cafeteria where a lot of people from all the different wings of the hospital came to eat. The staff would take Paula down there in her wheelchair and the speech therapist would work with her to relearn how to eat.

Imagine having to learn how to eat again. At dinner time, they had a group of head injury survivors; it was a mix of socialization and therapy. A therapist was there and they all ate together. I sat in the back and watched sometimes, but I usually used that time to go down and eat at the cafeteria downstairs.

I thought, "Wow, I'm here with you, Doug," but I don't remember thinking, "I'm getting better." I just knew that this is what's going on. Each day they would have me do things. I was working with my arms and my legs and my brain and playing with toys.

They kept me doing stuff. I didn't ever know if it was Sunday or any other day. They just came in and got me and took me to do what I needed to do.

When professionals refer to someone with severe head injuries, and I imagine with severe strokes, there is a phrase I heard, "They have a flat affect." That means the individual is awake, but not very interactive; they're not processing language and facial expressions normally. They have a distant stare and are in slow motion in a way.

That's another manifestation of those electricians rewiring stuff. Some of the more intense emotions and interactions just aren't back online yet.

I tried to make them happy. I wasn't working on making me happy. I wanted to make them happy. I'm sorry that I don't remember Doug much, but I remember Aik Teong would talk to me and would just be there. He brought me different books and read them to me. Doug's sister came by every day with her husband. I first remember feeling that I just wanted to make it okay with people. Not for me, but for other people. I wasn't thinking of me.

Friends came in, and I don't know how I was with them. Doug says that we had a birthday party for me. He took pictures of it and I have seen them. I sort of remember it, but not many of the details. Old friends from Connecticut and our navy days came to see me in Monroeville. It was really cool that people would come. Some of them made long trips to come, not just coming from right around there. That was cool. I don't remember any of the visits to the hospital in Ohio even now, though.

Paula never was greedy for anything for herself. She was always a giving person and still is. She gave to her friends and to her sister Maggie. She also probably gave over control of what the next step was to me, because she knew I was going to do it anyhow.

I don't remember that. I remember Doug taking me to therapy at the hospital once. I said, "You should've shot me. You should go on and live, I ain't worth it."

I told her I was out of bullets. She didn't say that in Monroeville. Quite frankly, she hadn't recovered enough to have that emotion.

She started having feelings that things hadn't gone how she'd wanted them to go pretty shortly after we came home after five months at HealthSouth. She was depressed. I made a sign for Paula's room that read, "Your recipe for recovery is three parts therapy and hard work, two parts good nutrition, one part rest and recreation, and ten parts patience." We had to reflect on that sign every once in a while when things weren't going as well as she or I wanted.

When we were at HealthSouth, they had a piece of equipment the therapists were using to get me to walk. They had me standing up and there were five people and a walker with my arm strapped in trying to get me to move.

It was a platform walker, a regular walker with a raised tray on the effected side that her arm could be strapped into. I was happily recruited as one of the folks working with her to help her learn to walk again. The therapists let me take charge of her right foot and slide it forward when it was time. Meanwhile, other therapists were making her body move like she was a wire figure in order to help her brain remember how to walk. This really seemed to amuse Paula. I remember her laughing a lot when she was trying to walk.

I thought it was funny that these people were doing all this stuff with me. It's nuts! It was funny and neat that they were doing that. Here at home when I go to therapy I tell the therapist, "I don't want to fall; you can rip my pants trying to keep me up." I've fallen with Doug and I go, "Oh shit." I just say, "Well, this is it. I don't complain about pain."

I remember in Monroeville, I got to where I could eat real food and that was wonderful.

My nephew sent her one of those big, stuffed Vermont Teddy Bears that come in a box with air holes. It's a really cool "Get Well" bear with a greeting card. It was wearing a chocolate bowtie. We opened the box and Paula held it for a little while and seemed to like it. When I went back to her room later, the chocolate bowtie was gone. I mentioned it to the nurses. Suddenly, it was like there was a fire; the nurses ran in looking all over for the chocolate bowtie that they had determined Paula was not ready to eat. They feared she might choke on it as she wasn't eating solid food yet. They even did an x-ray to find out if it was lodged in her throat. There was nothing there. She had eaten it and it turned out that she was fine. We had been pushing the hospital to allow her to start eating solid food. The chocolate bowtie was too great a temptation, so Paula took it upon herself to eat it without permission.

The teddy bear bow disappeared. I took it off and ate it, because I hated the food.

She loves chocolate. The speech therapist, a lovely girl, came in and was beside herself. I remember saying, "So, she can eat solid food now, right?" and she answered, "Well, I guess so!" They were going to perform a barium swallow test to check out her swallowing mechanics; another routine procedure for them. I had asked, "Why can't we just let her eat a cracker and see how it goes?" They told me that's not what they do. Turns out that is precisely what she did on her own. She was back on solid food the very next day, but she was carefully monitored for a week or more.

They gave me something to eat and I said, "Aaah! This is gross."

When she started eating normal food, we found out that her sense of taste was apparently not hooked back up yet either, since everything tasted horrible to her for at least a month.

Talking was a whole other matter. At HealthSouth, we learned about aphasia and apraxia of speech. Aphasia, caused by damage to the left hemisphere, is a language disorder in which individuals may have impairment in the ability to use or comprehend words. It can cause difficulty understanding words, finding the word to express a thought, understanding grammatical sentences, and reading or writing words or sentences.

Apraxia of speech is difficulty initiating and executing voluntary movement patterns necessary to produce speech when there is no paralysis or weakness of speech muscles. It may cause difficulty producing the desired speech sound or using the correct rhythm and rate of speaking. Paula had both; she had trouble remembering words and how to use them to form sentences, and making her vocal cords and mouth work to say the words. Having both must be one of the most frustrating things in the world.

We learned that everything else that requires action in your body has two pieces to it, too. The brain must first remember what to do and then also be able to tell the muscles or other system to do something if that system has been *reconnected* to the brain, except for the automatic actions like breathing and heartbeats. There's a connection between the two, but was Paula's connection still there? Her ability to speak returned very slowly over the course of a year.

I was terrible with names. I knew Doug, Clypso, Maggie, and Aik Teong. I thought, "Your name is what?" But Clypso was steady in my brain.

The reason for that, and it's still this way today, is that the piece of her left temporal lobe that they removed is evidently where names and proper nouns were stored. She has trouble with all words that are capitalized: cities, months, names, etc.

I sort of remember watching movies with Doug and Aik Teong on Doug's laptop. When I got cleared to go outside, they would have my wheelchair and push me around. There was an old house that we could go up to in the wheelchair. Doug would push me up the hill and down the hill and around the building. I remember how nice it was to be outside near trees again.

The hospital was on the end of a road so you didn't have to have so many people by you, which was nice. I could go out and to be outside and I just felt like, "Oh gosh, I'm outside!" I found trees that I could talk to.

# CHAPTER 10

# TWO STEPS FORWARD, ONE STEP BACK

Paula drove herself pretty hard. Her therapists and I also drove her. When she could come out of isolation, they moved Paula to a room about halfway up the hallway from the nurses' station; it was just the next available room after she was out of isolation. They started working her hard on day one and didn't slow down a bit until they discharged her to go back home to Ohio.

They had my room away from the nurse's station; they had me up near the end of the hallway. I don't know if I was driving them crazy or what. I remember being farther up the hallway, and I enjoyed that. Aik Teong read to me, he read me The Little Prince, which has always been very important to me. He would sit there and talk to me when I was awake, and then he'd just sit there and wait for me to come back. He would talk to me.

Doug was in there too, but he was taking care of all the problems and stuff, so I remember Aik Teong more. It was funny that he read me The Little Prince. I don't know if I asked him to do that or what.

The Little Prince is probably best described as a children's book that's meant for adults, too. It was written by a French author and is a really good book about just living. It's hard to describe.

Paula gave me a copy of it early in our relationship, after just a few dates, really. I think my reading, liking, and understanding it was sort of a test of my sensitivity and compassion. If I hadn't appreciated it, then Paula would have been less interested in me. Since I seemed to get it, I was okay.

When we met first, I gave Doug a copy of The Little Prince. If he'd come back and told me he wasn't very interested in it, I'd have said, "Nah." But he said, "Wow, this is really cool!" so I decided I'd keep him.

When Aik Teong read it to me, I thought, "Wow. Wow." He understood what it meant to me too, and wanted to read it to me for that reason. I don't know how long I kept with it each time he read it to me. I'm sure that it took a long time for him to read it to me while I was awake and alert, since I still took frequent naps.

In her early time there, Paula was drifting in and out of sleep. She was still *clearing* and the staff was working her hard. They started her therapy on day one; physical therapy, occupational therapy, speech therapy, and even recreational therapy. The contemporary theory on brain injury is that you need to get back in action as soon as possible because it helps the brain kick-start the reformulation process. It gets those electricians working to rewire the brain.

Plus, it keeps your body moving instead of just lying in bed and going to waste. I worked with people, with different therapists, and that was always fun. I enjoyed them. They were all different types of people but they were all good. They were focused on me and were happy to be able to work with me.

Paula was in the rehab hospital for about five months. The accident happened on February 9; she got to HealthSouth in early March and came home in August. I'm grateful that they worked her really hard.

She got up in the morning, had breakfast, went to one type of therapy, then had a small rest, and then went to another type of therapy. When dinner time rolled around, she was usually pretty tired.

I went to bed at 9:00, and I woke during the day. I really enjoyed the therapy.

Visiting hours were over at 8:00 p.m., but I normally left around 8:30 because after the first couple of weeks, I gave her a shower every night. I felt that was important, and it took a little bit of the load off the nurses, so they didn't mind me staying a little later.

He had to get me in the chair and roll me over to where you could get sopping wet, and he'd wash me very carefully.

She had quite a bit of swelling on the left side of her head because of the piece of her skull that was missing. The extra room gave the fluid in her brain somewhere to go without causing damage. The left side of her head swelled up to be about the size of a small cantaloupe, but that was okay because the skin swelled and provided structure to hold her brain together.

The survival mode was all about these weird procedures like the Greenfield filter. At HealthSouth, it was all about a whole different set of things and learning processes. I met a new kind of doctor that I never knew about; this is a doctor that everybody with a head injury or stroke will probably meet.

They are called physiatrists. I got to learn a lot more about the challenges of recovery from them.

Physiatrists are doctors that specialize in bringing people back from injuries of one sort or another. They are medical doctors, but they specialize in rehabilitative medicine of all sorts. Dr. Shymansky was wonderful.

There were a couple of physiatrists that were in charge of all the wings at HealthSouth, but Dr. Shymansky was the one that supervised Paula's care plan. She came and visited Paula at least every other day and made sure that the therapists were doing their jobs well.

During Paula's stay in the rehab hospital, her head swelled up significantly. We saw neurosurgeons and neurologists about it. One neurosurgeon that we went to suggested that she have a lumbar shunt installed, which is a drain in the bottom of the spine that drains out excess cerebral spinal fluid into the stomach cavity; this was a helpful procedure for her.

Her brain was still injured, but was healing and she was working hard. The fluid buildup in her head was an expected side effect of the injury. They would have liked for it to drain naturally, but it wasn't, so they put in the lumbar shunt. The next morning, her head looked like a deflated football because all the excess cerebral spinal fluid that had built up was gone.

Before the shunt, the left side of Paula's eye and head were swollen so much that her eyelid was pushed down a little bit. A day or two after they had the lumbar shunt put in, all the swelling went down.

Then, another problem cropped up—now she didn't have enough bone structure in her skull to hold her brain in place. Too much of her skull was missing and her brain was moving around slightly, which is not good. It turns out that one of the human body's strongest instincts is maintaining a stable focus on the world based on the position of the brain being centered and anchored. Paula's was neither. Her brain was actually moving around slightly in the new environments after the lumbar shunt was installed.

As a result of this movement, Paula developed what I learned was called midline shift syndrome. In layman's terms, this is what happens when your brain isn't anchored well in your body as a central reference point for all your senses and movement. Your brain is an anchor point for your whole world. If it doesn't have a consistent frame of reference, then vision, speech, and your whole body just slows down to counteract the constant shifting. The body and brain become sort of disconnected.

The way I understand it is that the body can't keep up with the moving brain and everything slows down to compensate; Paula got really groggy and tired and wasn't comprehending what was going on around her as much as she had been. It wasn't a life-threatening problem, like many of the things in the survival stage were. It was more like something that was hampering the rehabilitation, so we had to figure out what to do about it.

She didn't go back into a coma, but her body slowed down to the point that she was lethargic and couldn't communicate well. She also couldn't put in the work to get better, so it was a real problem. It was a big step backwards, and made us take new steps to get back on track. There were days when Paula wasn't ready for therapy, so they didn't try her. She doesn't remember that because she started getting groggier about halfway through her time at HealthSouth. It came on slowly, but we could definitely see that she was sleeping more. She was less interested in therapy and food.

We had been going to a new neurosurgeon in Pittsburgh since Dr. Markarian was a long way away in Akron. In addition, Dr. Shymansky had worked with him before, so it made sense to switch.

At one point, we all made the decision that it was time to put her skull back together. That week, I went back to Ohio to go to the office on Friday and take care of the horses like I had been doing. On Sunday morning, I went to the hospital to pick up the box with the pieces of her skull in it. I put it in the back seat of my car and headed for Pittsburgh. The neurosurgeon was scheduled to put her back together on Monday morning.

I had the missing piece of Paula's skull in a box with dry ice in the back seat of the car. I didn't know how long the dry ice would last, so I wanted to hurry to preserve the integrity of her bone, but I kept thinking, "What happens if the cops pull me over for speeding and ask what's in the box. I'd have to say, "A piece of my wife's skull!" I didn't think that would go well. They'd tell me to get out of the car and it would probably go downhill from there.

What I really wanted to do was to stop somewhere and carve my initials in the piece of her skull. After all, what guy wouldn't want to carve his initials in his wife's skull? I think you have to find humor wherever you can in times like this; however macabre that humor might be.

I made it safely back to Pittsburgh with the box and dropped it off at the hospital where they put it in their freezer. The neurosurgeon put her skull back together first thing on Monday morning. That was about four months after the accident. She was not awake much on Tuesday or Wednesday.

The neurosurgeon told me that this was to be expected, as her body and brain were getting used to another whole new physical arrangement and working relationship.

On Wednesday I got to the hospital around 9:30 a.m. I sat with her while she slept and talked to her when she was awake. I went to lunch around noon and came back to her room around 1:00 p.m. to find her non-responsive and shaking pretty violently. I didn't know what was going on, but I knew it didn't look good and was something I hadn't seen before. Paula had never done this before and I didn't know what it was or to be watching for it. I learned later that she was having a seizure. I didn't know to expect these. I was really frantic. Nobody had told me to expect seizures to develop.

I dragged the nurse into the room by the arm. Paula was seizing for the better part of two hours, which is a very long time. It can be a life-threatening thing. They put a peripherally inserted central catheter (PICC) line into a major artery in Paula's chest so they could pump drugs into it to manage the symptoms. That was challenging because she was shaking a lot when they were trying to do it and it took the doctors a long time to get it right. That was a bad day.

One of the things that people with moderate to severe head injuries will sometimes experience is seizures. Seizures happen because a part of the brain has the equivalent of scar tissue and the electrical connections are disturbed and get scattered. It's sort of like a lightning storm in your head. I am putting this in layman's terms because I don't understand all the medical/technical concepts. The part of the brain that was damaged doesn't send or receive electrical signals properly.

What they surmised happened is that when the skull was put back together, there was a new, very slight bleed in a part of the brain that gave rise to this new and disturbing development. I give the neurosurgeon some credit and don't fault him for it because he's doing some pretty fancy surgery. I'm not one of these people that sue others every time something doesn't go perfectly. That surgery is not a routine surgery, and where he worked was likely the focal point of the seizures.

That incident kicked off several years of seizures at random intervals. One of the things that I did to help diagnose them, which I suggest that you do if your loved one is recovering from a traumatic brain injury (TBI), is keep a log of seizure activity.

Record what time it started, what may have triggered it, how long it lasted, and a description of the symptoms. That helped the neurologist figure out how to treat them better. If you are prone to seizures, you've got to learn your triggers. Paula's triggers are exhaustion, excessive heat, and hunger.

We learned a very different set of symptoms to look for at HealthSouth than in the ICU in Ohio. The issues we had at HealthSouth probably weren't life-threatening, although I wasn't sure about the whole seizure thing.

My roommate, Sue, had gotten out of the hospital and gone home. Doug, Aik Teong, and I went to the ice cream place and then drove a long distance out to her house in the country. There was this barn and horses where she worked. I thought, "Wow! Cool!" Doug pulled up as she came out and opened the door. Then I went off into Never-Never Land.

Paula had a seizure right there at Sue's place. Seizures after a brain injury are pretty common from what we were told. It can be different for everybody; for Paula, it can also be caused by sensory overload. If she goes into a room full of people and everybody is talking, she begins to shut down because she can't process the inputs quickly enough.

She was not capable of recognizing when it was happening, so I would have to watch her and determine when it was time for us to leave. That continues to this day, although it has gotten somewhat better.

A lot of times when I would just go outside of the hospital to some of the places we would visit, I would go back in the room and go to sleep.

If people asked or stopped us to talk on the way back to the facility, I'd say, "Paula needs to lie down for a little while." She hasn't had what you would formally call a seizure now since 2006, which is awesome. She takes three different anti-seizure drugs on an ongoing basis. That's part of the art of neurology.

It took three years to find the right combination of drugs. It's hard to achieve the right balance of anti-seizure drugs because you have to bring them on slowly. You bring on a dose of an anti-seizure drug over the course of several weeks, increasing the dose a little bit at a time so as not to overload the body's ability to process the positive and negative effects. If you want to change it, you also have to decrease it very slowly and add the other one in very slowly. This period of time required very close coordination with her neurologist and careful adherence to the medication plan you develop with him/her. Really, you're almost like a chemist when you're mixing all the pills up for people to take. Then, you must watch and wait to assess the effectiveness of the new mix of drugs. When you're in that interim period, you don't know if they are going to have more seizures. And those are really hard to watch.

We did fun and special things whenever we could. When our friends from Connecticut came down, we brought a lobster dinner from Red Lobster into HealthSouth and we all ate in the conference room together. Paula enjoyed that a lot—well, as much as she enjoyed anything.

We had a birthday party for her and she blew out the candles. That happened at four and a half months, almost three-quarters of the way through her time at HealthSouth. She said she remembered things early on; there's a lot about Monroeville that she still doesn't remember. I feel it was all part of her therapy to be as engaged as possible. She was present for events and she participated.

The beauty of HealthSouth's treatment plan is that they treat you as normally as possible and always keep pushing you to take the next step toward normalcy. That drive to recover is what's really important there.

The nurses took time to come in and talk to me.

The nurse wasn't just zipping in and zipping out and taking vital signs. It seemed to me that the hospital took the approach of working together to get better, rather than allowing their patients to lie there waiting to get better. They believed patients would have a much improved outcome if they pushed and worked them and had everybody pushing in the same direction. We all pushed.

Paula is a person who is consistently eager to please other people. I think she was trying to make the therapists happy by getting better. I'm not at all sure that she was doing things for her own sake, but I didn't know this because she couldn't talk about that at the time.

When I got back to Ohio, I'd go to the therapy places and sit there and talk to anyone around. There was this one man sitting there and I said, "Hi, how are you?" He replied, "I'm fine," and I kept after him because he just looked sad. I asked him, "What do you want?" He said, "It would be very nice to get a cat." I asked him why he couldn't have a cat; surely he can have it inside. He said, "Could I have a cat?" That was a positive. He acted more positive after that and I felt like I helped him. But I didn't act that way to roommates and stuff.

Actually, she did. She tried with all her roommates to be friendly and challenge them and engage them.

After breakfast, the speech therapist took Paula down to the cafeteria where families and hospital staff were eating. She would eat with the physical therapist that was helping her relearn the mechanics of picking up a spoon, putting it in your mouth, and swallowing. It was a therapeutic lunch. Dinner was more social because they had a group of six or eight patients who were able to go down to a little room in the head injury wing and eat together.

I had breakfast in bed, lunch at the cafeteria, and then dinner in the room. That was the sloppy stuff, not normal food. When we finally got permission for Doug to take me for a drive, we would go down to the ice cream place.

When Paula stole the chocolate bow tie off the Vermont Teddy Bear, she still didn't have any sense of taste or smell and didn't want to eat. She lost a lot of weight; she had lost forty or fifty pounds in four months. One of the things that Aik Teong and I did was try to make her eat lunch because she needed the food to recover and the energy to do all the work that they were asking her to do. Half the time, she ended up wanting a peanut butter and jelly sandwich.

Doug had to eat so we would go into the cafeteria and I would have food from there. It was real food.

Paula's eating and swallowing skills had improved by that point. That was both good emotionally and also for rehab. She still didn't seem to have much of a sense of taste, so food still wasn't all that interesting to her.

Later in her time in Monroeville, we got permission to take her for car rides, so we would go out. She and Aik Teong and I would stop at an ice cream parlor that we liked and she did enjoy ice cream. Before this, we had only received permission to take her for rolls in the wheelchair, a nice, high-end wheelchair. We would start by just circling the building and going around the lot out in the trees.

Early in her recovery, she had no sense of taste or smell, so you can imagine that her appetite was light. If she had not wanted to eat ice cream, I would've taken her back to the surgeons and said, "There's something drastically wrong here; you missed a part of her when you put her back together!"

# CHAPTER 11

# GRINDING IT OUT:
# LOTS OF HARD WORK
# & SOME FUN

Three weeks in, we were starting to take Paula from the second floor down to the ground and outside. After dinner every night we would go down the hill and up another hill to an old historic house.

And being outside in Mother Nature was, like, wow!

It was pretty there and we would listen to the birds and sit and talk for a while. I'd roll her back and she'd take a shower, and then Aik Teong and I would leave.

I remember a friend named Lynne Anne Nanney. She came over from central Pennsylvania and took me out and rolled me around. We'd be in the parking lot and I thought that was cool that she did that.

Aik Teong and I tried to fill in the gaps of time for Paula during the hours that she wasn't with one staff member or another. I bought my first laptop computer and it had a DVD drive so we took it downstairs to the conference room and three or four times a week we'd have movie night. I'd rent a DVD and the three of us would sit there, eat microwave popcorn, and watch it on the laptop. Paula enjoyed that at the time, but she doesn't remember it. I understand.

I always thought it was funny that I remembered Clypso's name first; he's a horse. I remember I did a lot of ambulance trips.

There were lots of tests that needed to be run for Paula. At one point, the doctors thought that she had a blood clot in her leg. With the IVC filter in, it wasn't life-threatening because it would stop the clot from moving to her lungs or brain, but they wanted to find out for sure. I didn't have permission to drive her in the car yet, so every time she had to go to a doctor outside of the HealthSouth building, she was transported in an ambulance.

One of the key facets of her improvement in my mind was to constantly look for places where we could take Paula to challenge her and work her more. She was always up for it. It might have seemed tempting to let her rest and recover, but everything that I learned indicated that it was best to keep pushing.

Being an advocate under constantly changing rules of engagement was a challenge. I had to act as the coach as well as the advocate, looking regularly at where she's been, where she's at, and where we wanted to take her in the course of treatment and recovery. The players are on the field and somebody has to watch and plan the next moves, strategies, and actions. It takes a lot of effort, and for those who don't have the capacity or skill to be on the field of action, you can lose hope, and so can your loved one who is trying so hard to recover.

Nobody would let Paula lose hope, though she had some bad periods in Monroeville. She went through some times where she was depressed. Quite frankly, I saw that as positive because to me, it meant that she was becoming more aware of her reality. If you weren't upset and depressed about losing so much of your former self and your abilities, you weren't processing it thoroughly.

Later in Ohio, Doug would drive me to therapy and I would say, "Doug, I should die and let you go on and live, because I'm just dragging you down. I'm a pain and I can't do anything." I'd have moments like that where my brain went "Eeee!" and then it would be okay. Doug would put me in the chair and roll me up and later he'd let me walk up the stairs and I thought, "Cool! I can do that. I don't have to use the damn chair."

Dr. Shymansky, the physiatrist, talked about antidepressant drugs and I didn't really want to go there. I think modern medicine is too quick to push antidepressants. That's how I feel, so I resisted it. They didn't like that because they thought that was what we should do. I said, "Let's give it a week, or two, or three." And in those weeks, she did brighten up some. But when she came home, she had worse days because she was in a comfortable, familiar environment but she wasn't her old self.

I remember people and what they did—one lady came in and found us a corner in the cafeteria. She was my speech therapist and worked with me on my vocabulary. She was really a nice person. I would go in her office and she would find a place for us to sit. That was really cool of her. One lady had us play and there was a whole group of people and things and you were supposed to throw a ball. We'd have to throw a ball or do other stuff. We had to interact with people and that was cool.

Paula had social interaction focused on playing and rebuilding. I can't say enough good things about HealthSouth and their philosophy. They seemed to have an organizational philosophy that, "This isn't a place you go to rest and hope to get better, this is a place you come to work to get better." Everybody on the team seemed to share that vision, and all the therapists were great in that way. They were such caring and wonderful people.

I took her wedding ring over to a jewelry shop in the local mall in Monroeville and had it put back together. We got all Paula's jewelry back on her. Early on, I recall her saying, "Where's my bracelet? The one with the horses on it?" Getting Paula's jewelry back on was part of her becoming more normal.

# CHAPTER 12

# HOMECOMING:
# NOT THE DANCE, BUT A
# GREAT DAY NONETHELESS

After about four months, it was time to plan for Paula's homecoming. But I didn't know what I needed to do at home to modify it for her to be safe. It wasn't like she broke her leg and would come home in a wheelchair for a week before she could start taking showers again. This was very different because this would be a life-changing move for us both. We would never again live in our home the way we did before the accident. Planning for the next phase started to become really important, especially because we lived in a two-story house.

Our bedroom was upstairs at the time. We had steps to get in and out of the house, so it wasn't what you might call a handicap-accessible house. Most people don't have such a house; who thinks about such things in your younger years? I asked the occupational therapist at HealthSouth to come to the house, which was about two hours away. We did a walk-through and she acted as a consultant, telling me exactly what I needed to do to prepare for Paula's return, and told me how to prepare things with safety in mind.

It took almost a month for me to get the house ready for Paula to come home, since I was only working on it two to three days per week. HealthSouth wouldn't let her come until I said that I had done all the necessary preparations, even things like putting in a chairlift. Aik Teong and I put that in. We built a ramp from the deck around the side so that Paula could get a motorized wheelchair around to the outside from the back porch.

We put in a sidewalk where before we just had grass and things like that. We didn't have a hospital bed when Paula first came home. I found a place called Access to Independence nearby that had all sorts of different medical equipment and made arrangements to have a hospital bed at home. They gave us a free month to use the bed, and we ended up getting more necessary and useful items there like a tub seat, the bedside commode, and even a four-wheel outdoor mobility scooter. These folks were really great in helping me get the things we'd need to help Paula live in our house safely.

Another helpful thing the occupational therapist did was to give me a list of equipment that we'd need. Some of it the staff obtained for us in Monroeville, and we threw it in the back of the car and brought it home.

Some stuff we actually needed to test there at the hospital. They made Paula and I demonstrate together that we could do what we needed to do when professional caregivers were no longer a part of our 24/7 care. We showed them that we could get her out of bed and transfer her to a chair because she still couldn't stand when she first came home.

The hospital bed was necessary because she had been lying down at a slight angle for so long in rehab that suddenly being flat was excruciatingly painful. She laid at a slight angle to help improve her breathing and circulation during her stay at HealthSouth. We had to get a hospital bed and start off with that same angle and just lower it one notch a week for about a month until her body acclimated to lying flat in bed again.

I got to go home with Doug one day in early August, about six months after my accident. We just got in the car and he drove me home.

It was pretty awesome. Paula went from Akron to Monroeville in an ambulance, but when we left HealthSouth, she came home in a car - our car. It wasn't like getting a new puppy when she was coming home, bounding in and eager to explore her surroundings with speed. It was more like, "How are we going to get up these stairs again?" When we got home, we started the drive for normalcy.

At Monroeville, I'd have all these people and it was really cool. Then I get to our house, and it's Doug and Aik Teong; and then Ginny, a friend from Denver who came and stayed with us for three weeks shortly after I came home. Aik Teong stayed on until Monday for me.

Being home was another learning experience. I really came to appreciate all the stuff that Paula did before her accident, like cooking, because immediately I had to start taking care of Paula. That was my first priority, followed by other things like cooking, laundry, and cleaning the house. I actually went back to work fairly soon, too. We hired a home health care aide to make this possible.

The whole time Paula was in Monroeville, I continued to coordinate and supervise my interns. I usually taught two classes in marketing or management. My colleagues took care of much of my other work, but at any given time I was still responsible for supervising twenty or so interns in the real world outside our bubble of recovery. I worked virtually. Each student sent me a weekly journal.

While she was in Monroeville, I would read the journals, respond to them, and challenge them to think about this and that. My interns knew what was going on in our lives, but couldn't tell if I was working with them from my office at Mount Union or from Paula's room in HealthSouth. The college appreciated me still supervising my interns. It gave me some sense of normalcy, too. Sometimes, when Paula was off with the speech therapist (who didn't want anybody else in the room), I'd be working with my interns.

That may be why I saw Aik Teong a lot, because he had nothing to do other than read and Doug had all this stuff to do.

For the first several weeks at home, I had to do some strange things I had never been aware of before. I had to learn how to give Paula injections. I thought, "I have to do what?" For the first three weeks after she came home, she had to have a daily anti-clotting shot in her stomach because those who are less mobile have an increased chance of forming blood clots.

The hospital staff taught me how to give her a shot. I had to help her use a bedpan when she had to go to the bathroom at night. I had to help her take showers. I had to help her to the bathroom during the day when she was downstairs. In short, I had a lot going on.

A lot of times, he had to change the bed because I peed in the bed at night. I'd think to myself, "Why can't you turn over for him?!"

For months, there were accidents and I had to deal with changing the bed at night. Paula felt worse about some of this than she did about many other issues with her recovery.

But Doug would have to work, work, work. I would go to bed at 9:00 and he'd take me and put me in the bed and then go downstairs and do lots of other things.

Most of the time after Paula went to bed; I'd go downstairs, do the dishes and clean a little bit. I learned a lot of caregiving tips during our time at HealthSouth that really helped us a lot at home.

I learned about the concept of driving toward recovery there and continuing to do so.

Before we could move back home, we needed to put together a whole new medical team. We had to go out and find the doctors and therapists, evaluate them, and make sure that they were good. I had started doing this at HealthSouth. I had appointments set up and HealthSouth helped a lot with that.

They had a checklist: "Who's your neurologist there? When's your next appointment?" I had initial intake appointments set up during the first two weeks after we got home.

I felt like I was putting a baseball team together and picking the skill players for each position. That's not a bad analogy to use, as you do want the best person at each position so the whole team (including your loved one) can be successful. If one of your players isn't performing up to your expectations, you have to cut them and find one who will.

We found a neurologist and a physiatrist. It turns out there was a good physiatrist at our local hospital; they do a lot of geriatric care. Dr. Karen Gade at the hospital in Alliance is a very good physiatrist, and we also ended up going to Paula's original neurosurgeon, Dr. Markarian, because he was nearby in Akron and we really liked him.

We went to all the initial appointments with the new doctors and therapists. The only one that didn't work out was a neurologist in Massilon, Ohio that someone recommended to me. We had to fire him after the initial appointment and find a second neurologist. Dr. Al Jaberi, the new neurologist, turned out to be another great doctor and a wonderful human being.

We also had appointments with all the therapists that she needed. When we started, we were going to three different kinds of therapy three or four days a week in two different locations, in addition to doing all the therapy at home. Occupational therapy was in one place, working primarily with her arm and activities of daily living, like taking a shower. We had a physical therapist in town who was a really nice lady who worked wonders for Paula. We also had a good speech therapist at the hospital.

She gave me a word puzzle activity book and I was supposed to read it, but I got ticked off. I didn't like those because they were too difficult.

I asked the therapists what I could do to help keep her moving forward. One of the things I did when Paula came home was to put her computer on a hospital table—one of those tables that go up and down beside the bed. She was in a high-end wheelchair that leaned back and had footrests so it was comfortable for her. It was a wheelchair designed for paraplegics, with a gel seat because we anticipated that she would have to use it for some extended period of time.

When I wheeled the computer up to her, she didn't remember how to turn it on. We started her training by simply learning how to turn it on, and when it booted up, I loaded Microsoft Word and said, "Okay, type the alphabet."

These were the things that I talked about with her speech and occupational therapists. It took her two-and-a-half weeks and many utterances of the word *shit* (that was one of the first words that she could remember) to type the alphabet. Whenever she ran into a wall trying to find a word, "Shit! Shit!" was what would come out.

Words weren't coming out, but somehow "shit" could. It seemed that when she got tired of trying to find or say the words she was looking for; she'd fall back on that old reliable expletive.

Paula started singing before she could even talk. The whole time in rehab, she could sing songs from beginning to end, even when she couldn't say the lyrics. I learned that brain scientists think that singing and poetry use different parts of the brain than speech does, so people who can't talk can often sing or recite poetry.

Early on in her time in HealthSouth, we'd be in the waiting room for an MRI or something and Paula could sing, "I Knew an Old Lady Who Swallowed a Fly." She could sing in perfect pitch, in perfect pronunciation, but she couldn't say the words without singing them.

There was a poem that she knew throughout her whole life, "The Owl and The Pussycat." She didn't know it after the accident, but we relearned it. That was one of the things we worked on at home. She memorized it again. It took her a week or so to relearn it. She can repeat it from start to finish to this day. She still has trouble with some other aspects of speech, particularly with capitalized words.

Then I lost that ability to sing.

Paula didn't lose her ability to sing, but she started to regain the ability to speak normally. As she progressed in her speaking, it became less important to sing and she just didn't do it.

When she could complete the alphabet on the computer in under an hour, I'd say, "Now for every letter, type an animal's name, or a food." I used common categories that I thought would be easier first steps. After a while, I introduced her to Microsoft Paint, a really basic drawing program, and she started drawing on the computer.

I'm not an expert, but I think those visual design efforts used different parts of her brain and contributed to her healing. Her neurosurgeon thought it was good cognitive and emotional therapy, too. Drawing was a good thing for her to do. Her art really developed. We got her a couple of better drawing programs later and she really took to them, even after being frustrated by having to learn all new commands and techniques.

Her art started to develop nicely and before long, actually, a few months, she was creating some lovely drawings. They were tribal in nature, like the Kokopelli-style drawings. As time went by, she was drawing pictures we used on our holiday cards and even ones that we had embroidered on shirts.

At first it was, "Ehhh," and then I could get to where it was nicer lines.

Interestingly, her new neurologist liked to see her drawings because it gave him good benchmarks by which to track her cognitive progress. This one was a horse lover from Syria whose family raised the old line of Arabians that raced across the desert, like in the movie Hidalgo. He didn't race, but he said that other members of his family did. He and Paula would talk horses for thirty minutes and then maybe talk a little bit about medicine. He's a sly fox, because that was cognitive analysis in a way, too.

He was tracking Paula's progress through her drawings. He'd look at them and say, "That's really pretty, but let me tell you what that means." I remember one time, he looked at a new drawing and he said that her ability to start using more complex color combinations indicated that certain neural connections were coming back online, being restored. I don't know neurophysiology and I don't know art, but I know what I like and I liked hearing that.

# CHAPTER 13

# SETTLING IN AT HOME & MOVING FORWARD AGAIN

One of the words that I heard a lot along the road to Paula's recovery, surviving, and driving, was plateau. One popular theory in head injury and strokes is that you get back all the abilities you can expect to get back within a year. Then you plateau.

It's interesting, but I'm not quite sure that it's true. We continue to see improvements. To this day, friends and family that visit once or twice a year tell me that Paula's made some progress again.

The issue is that progress is not a linear function. It's not a straight line. It's what's called a power function, an upward sloping curve. The curve flattens out with time, but there are still improvements to be gained. I think this becomes more evident as we learn more about the brain.

Doctors used to think brain cells didn't reproduce and now people think they do reproduce and rebuild. Obviously, they rebuild. Now, doctors use the term plasticity to refer to the brain's ability to rebuild and reconnect things.

One of Paula's dear friends lived with her husband in Denver, Colorado at the time. We'd met them in Guam in our navy days and became friends with them there. Shortly after Paula came home, I got a call from Ginny asking if she could come stay with us for three weeks to help us out during Paula's first weeks at home. We gratefully accepted and she came about a week later. Her time with us was really great. Paula enjoyed spending time with her and it helped a lot in our transition. Ginny assisted wherever she could and really was a godsend. Many families are in a position to have a family member come to stay and help.

We were fortunate to have great friends. The fact that we didn't have children presented a less complicated situation than for many other individuals who are recovering and raising children simultaneously. Having an older child or two would have helped, though, since they could have done some of the work around the house.

I was able to accomplish lots of other things while Ginny spent time with Paula. She was a tremendous help, but kind of poo-pooed it, saying, "Nah, this is no big deal," and I told her, "Yeah, it is a big deal." She had come from a long way to help and was giving Paula a lot of her time and attention - and letting me attend more to things around the house and at work. It was a very loving and caring act on her part.

Ginny is an organized, methodical person. She used to be a physical trainer, so she understood the mechanics of the body. She went with us to our first neurology appointment with the doctor we had to fire. There were three of us there to hear what the doctor had to say. The first appointment is always an intake assessment. It's not so much a treatment, but a chance for the doctor to get to know you and where you are so they can determine the most appropriate course of treatment.

This was a lesson learned that others can hopefully learn from as well. You need to approach that first appointment knowing that treatment won't happen then and there. They are going to talk to you, evaluate the patient, and then develop a treatment plan.

The first neurologist we went to checked out okay when I looked at his references. Paula was in a wheelchair and still had that flat affect. Her personality was dull and she didn't react to things much. She couldn't move her right side, couldn't talk, and still couldn't do a lot of things. She was still sitting in a wheelchair, as she couldn't walk without using a platform walker with lots of assistance.

The neurologist tested her for about ten minutes. He tested her ability to taste by giving her dabs of different flavored liquids on her tongue and determined that she could taste sugar but not salt or bitter yet. Those would come along later. After a few minutes of testing, he stopped and said, "This is about where you're gonna be."

I was so flabbergasted that I couldn't even smack him. I was floored. Ginny was floored. Paula was affected by it, but not as much. I was glad that she wasn't totally aware. He said that to her in the wheelchair when she couldn't even move.

I always told Paula that when she could get her right foot back up to crotch height, we'd go visit him again. If I got the chance, I'd tell him that he needed to be careful what he told patients because some of them might believe him! I guess that's why they call it practicing medicine. Some doctors never get good at it, but most do.

Before we could go back and give him our personal feedback, he moved down to Miami to treat geriatric patients.

Needless to say, we fired him immediately and found another neurologist in Canton, Ohio who turned out to be what we needed and were looking for. He didn't necessarily buy into that plateau theory, and neither did we. He was (and is) a great doctor and an awesome person. He even gave me his home phone number in case we had problems or questions. We didn't need to use that number often, but on the few occasions we did, he responded immediately, professionally, and compassionately. I didn't abuse that privilege because it's a real honor. The few times that I did call, he knew I needed answers. When Paula would have a seizure and I was a little concerned, I might call him for advice and reassurance.

That was an amazing thing. That's when you know you have the right kind of doctor and that they are part of the team. Paula lovingly refers to him as her "druggie" because one of his biggest tasks was to manage her seizure medications.

He was trying to find drugs that would balance me. Several times he had me change. Maybe this drug is not as mean or as hard as the other ones; maybe it's easier, but does the same thing. He would talk to Doug and they would start me on something, so we did the changes.

He always scheduled my appointments for the last time slot before lunch or the last one of the day. We'd talk about horses for a little while each time. Doug said it was more like twenty minutes when he'd ask if we needed to get around to talking about medical things.

He and I would write out very detailed transition plans between drugs, and it really became a lot to keep track of.

Both her neurosurgeon and the neurologist were highly trained specialists and very caring individuals. They both played major roles in Paula's physical and emotional recovery.

With this neurologist, we were struggling with the drug cocktail because Paula was still having three to five seizures a week. They were short in duration, from thirty seconds to a minute. They weren't grand mal seizures. They were more moderate. There are so many different terminologies for seizures and they change from time to time.

A seizure is a very scary thing to watch. I'd never seen one before Paula had her first one in the hospital after having her skull put back together. Everybody has triggers for seizures that are different and their manifestation is going to be different. I imagine that for some people, a hand might start twitching. You have to find that signal and be ready. It took a month for me to figure that out.

In Paula's case, she would lose the ability to talk just prior to a seizure. First, she'd lose most of her words and then not be able to say anything. Then, the right side of her lip would curl up. When that happened, I knew she needed to sit down or be in a safe position, because the next thing that would happen would be a seizure. Surprise seizures are no fun, but if you see her lip curl up, then you can get into that, "Okay, it has started raining, so let's close the windows," mode. I hate to say it becomes routine, because I still don't like that word.

It becomes more understandable and manageable. There were and still are times when she comes close and does not seize; she'll lose her words but never has the lip curl that marks crossing over what is known as the seizure threshold.

The neurologist taught me about the concept of a seizure threshold. If certain things push you above that line, then you're apt to have a seizure. Paula's seizure triggers seem to be exhaustion, heat, and hunger. They lowered her seizure threshold, or pushed her brain activity above it. I'm not sure how that works, but she'd cross the line and have a seizure.

One of the interesting things is that Paula was having, and still to this day has, what I call neurological transients. This may not be a valid medical term, but it works for me. Her ability to speak changes during the day. Sometimes I think she might be hungry so I ask her if she's hungry and she has a little something to eat and then her speech improves. Or, if she's tired, I might suggest a nap and she's better afterwards.

Our house in Ohio was modeled after an old farm house. It had a central core and rooms that went around that core, so you could walk all the way around the core of the house. We did a lot of therapy activities at home. Paula had a platform walker, so we walked around that core and tried to add one lap every couple of days.

The platform walker was a standard granny walker with an elevated tray for her right arm. I'd strap her arm into that tray before she walked. I'd walk behind her, holding on for dear life (or my dear wife). It was about a fifty-foot walk around the core of our house; it might take her five minutes to get around it, but we'd walk it after dinner every night and sometimes during the day if she wasn't too tired from her therapy sessions.

The team that we put together for Paula was pushing her; because that's the kind of team we wanted. I asked them what I could do at home to help. She was doing squat thrusts on a Total Gym exercise machine. There were workbooks with word puzzles and fill-in-the-blanks that the speech therapist used in the office. We bought three or four of them from a place in Akron. She could do those on her own. Paula took to doing stuff like that just the same as she took to all the therapy. She leaned into it and worked really hard on it.

We'd try to replicate and reinforce things Paula was doing in therapy at home. She would stand at the kitchen counter with her good hand up on it and do a sidestep. The walker moved forward, and eventually we had her walk backwards a little bit, but she could only do that on the linoleum, not on the carpet. It was good that she was changing flooring surfaces around the house. The one thing I couldn't do at home (and still can't) is occupational therapy. It seems to be more specialized and needs a location with people and equipment dedicated to it. More importantly, I think it requires an experienced touch to know how far to push a particular movement without doing harm.

He's not brave enough.

We added things in. I would ask the therapist, "If we had this set up so that it looks like this, is it safe for her to unload the dishwasher?" At some point early on, Paula started unloading the dishwasher. She'd put the dishes on the counter while sitting in her wheelchair. Then, she'd stand up and sidestep along the counter about six feet, moving the dishes along with her in increments. Then, she'd put them up in the cabinets and drawers. She was leaning on the counter, but standing up and working on improving her balance and strength. That was good for her balance and self-esteem, because she was helping now, plus working on muscles and controlling them at the same time.

He'd roll me in and when he did, I saw he had left everything on the counter. He'd go and get his cereal, but it should have been put up. I told him he needed to clean it up.

For me, it was easier not to have to get the cereal back out onto the counter the next day; we're going to eat that anyhow. The yard was a mess because I didn't do any weeding for about eight months. When we got home, I had an old tractor seat and some wheels from an old gas grill, so I built a little wooden frame for this tractor seat that sat about six inches off the ground for Paula to sit on and weed a little section of garden outside.

I had one of these big market umbrellas that you have on your patio furniture with the heavy base. I'd take the umbrella out, set it up in the yard next to a planter, lower Paula into that seat, and she'd push herself to pull weeds. The umbrella kept the sun off her. The first day she did that, she weeded a whole foot of garden and she was wiped out. The dogs were with her out there and they'd come up and nuzzle her - that's probably another reason she didn't get much weeded. She loves being out in the yard weeding, as she always did, and I found it fairly ironic that she was hollering at me for not keeping up with the weeds. I told her, "Well, you know, I'm kinda busy. Why don't you get to it? If you don't like 'em, go pull 'em."

# CHAPTER 14

# MORE STEPS FORWARD, SOME STEPS BACK... AGAIN

We learned that family members acting as caregivers are always going to be more conservative and paranoid than they probably need to be and certainly much more than the person being cared for is comfortable with.

Part of the challenge is letting somebody do something that is marginally unsafe if it has therapeutic value. On the other hand, the survivor is always going to be more risky than they need to be. In some ways, I was a friend, a husband, and a father to Paula. She really resented the father role where I had to make hard decisions that she didn't agree with, but were based more on safety than her being comfortable or happy.

The elaborate dance that takes place involves finding the overlap between what she feels like doing and what I think is safe and therapeutic. Those are two important terms and balancing the two became a challenge after Paula came home from HealthSouth, and even more important as she continued to improve.

She had osteopenia (weak bones) from not bearing much weight through her bones, so if she fell, there was a good chance she was going to break something. One morning, almost exactly one year after she came home, she fell at the bottom of the stairs while turning to get into her wheelchair. I made her stay still on the floor to take stock of things and see what, if anything, hurt. "Are you okay? Sit there and feel things and tell me if you're okay." She told me that her upper leg hurt but it was okay. When I got her up in her wheelchair; she was grimacing. She has an amazingly high pain threshold. I know if she grimaces, she's in a lot of pain.

I asked her again if it was okay, and she replied, "Yeah, it's okay. I can eat breakfast." She ate sitting in her wheelchair, and halfway through breakfast, she started feeling worse, so I told her I was calling an ambulance. She said, "No, no, it's okay." But I called an ambulance and they came and took her to the hospital - it turned out she had broken her hip and had to have surgery to put it back together with some metal pieces and screws. She was laid up for a little bit with that and it set her back on the therapy plans, or at least changed the focus for several months.

I don't remember that.

Paula wanted to do many different things that I thought were not safe and beneficial. Something like sitting out in the garden and weeding was very beneficial—emotionally, physically, and spiritually—but it wasn't easy getting her up and down. I had to deadlift her up and down in that little chair I made for her. It was probably not safe for me, and is probably one of the reasons my back isn't as good as it used to be.

But that's okay, it comes with the territory. You invest in things that are marginally less safe because they have therapeutic value. As an example, she wanted me to teach her how to butt scoot up and down the stairs to the basement. We designed our new house in North Carolina so she could drive her scooter around and walk in the door. I said, "Where's the value in scooting?" We haven't worked on that and she has understood that we weren't going to do it.

When I got to use my scooter, I was weed whacking and I wanted to have a radio, and so I walked up the stairs on the porch and the outlet where you could plug it in was down below, so I sat down on the step and plugged it in. All was cool, and then I went down the steps, but the handrail was too high. I was sitting there going, "Uhhh." So I called the neighbors on my cell phone and asked if they could come over and help me, and they came over and got me up.

I made sure Paula always had a phone with her. This incident is indicative of many other events like this. One of the reasons I believe Paula recovered to the degree she has is that she's one of the most stubborn, ornery people I've ever met in my life. That gave her the drive to do her part. If she hadn't been stubborn and ornery, we might not be having this conversation, because she might not have survived. From my observations, it seemed that her motivation during her therapy sessions was partially to please other people (her therapists) and partially to recover as much physical and cognitive function as she could.

Initially, when I wanted to go back to work, we hired a nurse's aide. I found out that dependent care was tax deductible, so it made it more acceptable financially, too. The aide sat there and slept sometimes while Paula was working on the computer, but they were good together. She made meals, talked to Paula, and made sure that she was safe while doing things like going to the bathroom.

I could use the potty in the powder room. It was always, "Lift Paula and put her on the potty. Lift Paula and sit her in the chair."

At some point it became possible for Paula to be home alone for a short time. There were certain things that were mandatory for her to be able to do in order to be home alone, so we worked on getting her to be able to do those things on her own. We had a powder room downstairs. At first, we figured out a way for her to drive her wheelchair up to the door of the powder room. I would have to go in with her and we'd have to do a little dance, with me holding her up while she moved her feet and turned to sit on the toilet. Soon we put a grab bar in and she was able to lower herself down and lift herself off the toilet. When she could stand up and shuffle from the doorway to the toilet on her own, she started using the bathroom on her own, which was good for both of us.

All that therapy we were doing, all that sidestepping at the sink and walking around was building her capabilities for improvement. We had that aide for several months, but then she progressed to where I felt it was safe for her to be home alone. But I didn't want her to be out of communication, so we got her one of those Life Alert systems with a button that she wore around her neck.

Paula got an electric wheelchair that she could use in the house in late 2002. Later, we bought a four-wheel outdoor mobility scooter for her. She could use this one to go check the mail and even visit some of our nearby neighbors. Early in 2005, three years after the accident, there was one occasion where she fell out of her scooter outside. She was out weeding in the scooter and fell out of it. So, she used the button.

I was trying to pull weeds out of the bushes and there were some sticky weeds and I fell out. I thought, "Shit."

Her glasses cut into her forehead and gave her a nasty, bleeding cut. It wasn't a deep gash, but facial cuts really bleed.

I was still lying on my face and I pressed the button and said, "I need a little help." The service said, "Do you want us to call your husband?" And I said, "No, and don't call an ambulance." The lady said, "Well, could we call some neighbors?"

I had arranged with a neighbor to be on call.

I was still on my face. I said, "Yeah, call Joan." While I was waiting for Joan, I turned myself up and I was leaning against the scooter. I heard her drive down the driveway and she couldn't see where I was sitting. I heard her stop and I said, "Okay, you're gonna come around and I'm a little weird, so don't freak out." She came around and I had a bloody shirt and bloody glasses, and she said, "Oh, I'll tell ya! What do we have to do?"

She probably asked Paula if she should call me and Paula probably told her not to.

I told her, "I need to get back into my scooter, do you think you can lift me?" She did, and halfway up, we had to rest because I was heavy. She got me in the scooter, and I asked her, "Can you bend my glasses so they're sort of straight and clean the blood off?" I took my scooter and went around to the porch where my indoor wheelchair was and I moved to that one.

After we went back inside, she asked what she could do and I said, "Can you wash my face off a little bit?" We did that, and then I asked her if she could go upstairs and get me another shirt. I took my shirt off and put a new shirt on, and she said, "What do I need to do now?" and I told her, "Oh, nothing. I'm okay."

The ambulance never did have to come. I found out about this episode when I came home that night. It was just like any other day, but there was a wet t-shirt in the utility tub. It didn't have any blood on it; she'd cleaned it all off. It looked like she had a forensic cleanup team or something. I asked Paula, "What's this all about?" She replied, "Oh, nothing." I looked at her face. Her glasses were still crooked and she had this gash on her forehead. It wasn't bleeding anymore, but I asked, "What happened?"

So she told me the story piecemeal. I have no doubt that Paula could write a whole chapter in this book of things she did that I don't know about, and wouldn't be particularly happy about her doing. It's a balancing act, a negotiation. To this day, there's not a day that goes by that I don't wonder in the back of my mind what could happen if I leave for more than an hour.

Being home alone is good for Paula. It's good for me. We need some time alone. Moreover, it's part of thriving and being normal. I still worry about seizures, even though she hasn't had one for many years now.

The last seizure she had was in 2006, the day we bought the piece of land in North Carolina where we currently live. It was a hot summer day in July and we were driving around in my car. We had been out looking at property and heat was one of her potential seizure triggers. It was our anniversary, July 23. The realtor's wife needed his car, so I offered to drive. When we were out driving around with the air conditioner on, we heard a loud thud, and then the dashboard started vibrating. Our air conditioning had stopped working and it started getting warm.

We went to look at two more pieces of land with the windows open, but it was getting too warm. We were camping in our motor home over on the other side of town, so we went back into the air conditioning there. But Paula had gotten too hot in the meantime and had a seizure that afternoon. That was her last one, thankfully, but we do realize that it may not be the last one she ever has. We did buy the piece of land, though. That allowed us to really start planning for the next part of the book - thriving.

We'd looked at the place first, and I'd said, "This is it! This is cool." We went back to the office and signed the contract to buy the property. They took it and we went back home and it went on from there.

The stress and the heat of the day probably triggered that seizure. Later, I took the squirrel cage blower out of the air conditioning and there was a dead mouse in there. That's what had happened. I removed it, put it back together, and it worked fine after that.

We continue this dance of mutual understanding to this day. As the caregiver, you don't want anything bad to happen to your loved one. You don't want them to take any risks, whether they're necessary or unnecessary. You do that out of love, but it's shortsighted. Letting people take risks, if they're reasonable risks, is beneficial because it's part of the process of continuing to thrive and recover. It may be what causes the little incremental gains in the future. If you get to a point where you quit trying, then you probably won't have more gains. Paula continues to try to do things, and she continues to try my patience.

There's a caregiver and then a husband. Doug was more of the caregiver than the husband. Before, when we went shopping, I would get out of the car and walk around without waiting. Now...

Early on, when we went shopping, we had a wheelchair outside the car and Paula got in the wheelchair and we took her in the store that way. It was hard for me to go shopping. She'd have to be in bed and I'd go grocery shopping or she'd sit in the car and wait and I'd have the air conditioning going.

That was when she was still having accidents, so she had a pad under her in the car. As soon as she could, after her walking got better, she would come in with me. Either we pushed the wheelchair in or I got a cart in the grocery parking lot, and she held on with the left hand and gripped with the right hand. She would walk behind the cart and walk through the store. It would take us almost forty-five minutes just to get milk, bread, and a few other basics.

I would make problems because I would throw my foot too far. I would think, "Wow. Oh look, cereal! I was so excited about walking around a store and looking at things that I would lose focus on walking.

We were spending more time thinking about her process than what we had to buy in the store, which was good. It was useful. Even today, Paula says, "Why don't we walk around the grocery store?" I suggest that maybe we don't need to do that because she's moved on past that. She walks on her own around the house, so she can jolly well drive the little store scooter around and see things.

I broke my hip and they put me in the wheelchair, and told me, "You need to walk," and that was ten years ago.

When I broke my leg later, they put me in a lightweight transport wheelchair scooter, so I could pull myself around the house using my legs and feet. This helped me to strengthen my leg muscles, which also helped my balance and walking ability when I could put more weight on my leg. I thought, "Why the hell didn't they give me a wheelchair where I have to move my feet doing that?"

That's something we may have missed out on.

That is something very important. If your legs don't work well, get a dang transport wheelchair and try to pull yourself around with your legs.

Or we could have mixed them; if you sit in a powered wheelchair and use that as your mobility, it doesn't help your mobility. In 2012, Paula broke her right lower leg and had to have a rod put in. She broke it in another one of those moments that I heard about where she was doing something she shouldn't have been doing.

Paula really doesn't like talking about this because she doesn't like getting caught, which I understand. She broke her leg, and she was non-weight bearing, so I got her a lightweight transport wheelchair. It's a foldable wheelchair you can throw in the back of your car. I had to push her around the house, she couldn't use it yet. So when she got to be weight-bearing again, she started pulling herself around, using her feet and legs.

Even to this day, Paula has that transport chair in the bedroom and in the morning and at night, she pulls herself out to the kitchen using both feet. So it's another kind of therapy that helps her work on her hamstrings just by pulling herself around with her legs.

But if I'd started earlier, I would've put more pressure on my right side. I'm sitting in the scooter with my stupid legs down there not doing a dang thing. Anything you can do, if you can do it, like moving your arms or moving yourself or your legs—it's exercise. I'm very mad that I didn't do that earlier.

We used to do mostly me in my scooter or Doug pushing me. But it wasn't my work and I'm very sad that I wasted those years of working.

She has made a lot of gains in other ways. But her hamstrings would have been stronger, for sure.

When I was living in the scooter, my foot was not doing a darned thing. Just sitting there.

Pedaling on a good floor exerciser is just as good, if not better than that. She gets bored, but the therapists say it's better exercise for your legs and brain if you do it right. All those body systems still have to be worked individually. Paula has computer things that she does every day, including a free online game called Daily Diff. It has two pictures side-by-side with ten differences that you have to find. Paula does that every morning and she also does word searches and jigsaw puzzles online.

These are very good programs.

It would be great if Paula would read more, whether it be books, magazines, or even billboards. She used to read a lot of books, but always at night while lying on her side in bed. She doesn't see therapeutic value in sitting around during the day reading a book, even though it would be very good for her cognitive processes. It would be great exercise for her mind. It's every bit as important as exercising in a wheelchair or going to occupational therapy. Paula has trouble accepting this, and I understand that, so I don't push it too hard. It's frustrating, too, because she can only read a little bit at a time. Reader's Digest helps with that. The stories are shorter, so she can read one and feel good about it.

I would go sit on the toilet and read Reader's Digest. But at first I couldn't read a whole dang sentence. I couldn't read anything. I just turned pages. Then I got to where I could read the jokes. Then I got to where I could read longer stories, but I had to put a liner underneath. I would start to read things in Reader's Digest, but if it was something about a horse, I would read the whole damn novel.

# CHAPTER 15

# CONTINUING TO CLIMB
# THE MOUNTAIN

As Paula got better, the challenge was that she got more selective in what parts of her recovery she wanted to push. This is uncomfortable for her to hear, even today, but it's the truth. I understand that she wants to be out working in the yard pulling weeds and planting things. She does this a lot. I worry about black widow spiders and copperheads and her not wearing gloves. She doesn't think or worry about these things as much as I'd like her to. We continue to work on these things.

The challenge is to get her to want to do more things like reading books. She prefers to be physically active. We have an exercise machine that sits on the floor, a fairly high-quality foot peddler exercise machine. I had this screwed to the floor so that it wouldn't move, and Paula could sit there and pedal.

The more she pedaled, the more she was firing all those little muscles and nerves that control all those different parts of her leg and foot movements. It's a good thing to help her brain, nerves, and muscles communicate and work together.

At first, we would have to tie her right foot to the pedal to keep it from falling off. Then she graduated to the point where she could pedal without her foot having to be strapped onto the pedal. It fell off occasionally, but she'd put it back on and keep going. She was pedaling just like she was on a bike. This showed that all the muscles in her leg and foot, big and small, were getting stronger and communicating with her brain again. Her therapist and I think it's better for her to retrain her brain and body than to pull herself around in the wheelchair. That's only one motion, whereas pedaling is many motions. Both are important.

I have to be lined up. If I sit too much, then I'm not lined up.

She has to keep adjusting her posture, which is also part of the benefit. Unfortunately, and this will probably come up in anybody's case, it's very boring to sit there and pedal. I understand that. With therapy in general, and specifically with brain injuries, an important part of the recovery process is that brain-eye-muscle feedback loop.

Your mind has to be paying attention, and when you're pedaling, the best thing to do would be to feel what your foot is doing so that the feedback loops reinforce those brain-muscle pathways. If you consciously think, "My foot slipped this way," you benefit. If you're distracted, you get only a partial benefit.

Even if it is boring, we're okay with it. Paula will call friends and talk to them on the phone while she's pedaling because it's more fun, but it's less therapeutically valuable.

But I'm listening and sensing my foot staying on or off. I know that it's going around and I think, "How is this foot doing all the work, not the left foot?"

Doing something else while pedaling does dilute the overall effectiveness of the exercise, according to her therapists. But we'll accept the small loss of benefit if she does it more often.

Every head injury is different. Early on in Ohio, I found a brain injury support group that was made up of brain injury survivors and their family members or their loved ones. We went to a couple of meetings and I found them useful, but Paula really didn't like them. They had ice cream and they might have had a speaker present on one topic or another.

Some of the brain injury survivors were pretty negative and upset, and they seemed to be satisfied with where they were. They didn't seem to share Paula's perspective of always improving. Paula didn't find them that useful. The time commitment to go to one meeting twice a month was more than I needed unless we were both getting something out of it. On the other hand, I already had a very supportive network of people at work.

Another part of getting back to normal included getting Paula's skull worked on, since it had some bumps, extra holes, and a few missing pieces. It was not as much of a physical improvement as it was emotional. We went to a well-known plastic surgeon that did microsurgery. They surgically filled in the holes with titanium mesh and something like a bone concrete. The bone concrete resembles Plaster of Paris, but it grows a matrix of little channels in it and the blood vessels and nerves grow back through it, it's like artificial bone. As part of the preparation, they took a 3-D CT scan of her skull. I saved this image on her computer. It's a 3-D, rotating image of her skull and is one of the weirdest things I've ever seen.

She's got several square inches of that regrown bone in her head now. She had a flap of skin that went right down the center of her skull where her hair parts that still has a small dent in it; that was too close to her eye socket and they couldn't rebuild that section.

She's still got a few extra holes in her head; one time she had a little bit of internal pressure building up, so she went back in the hospital and the neurosurgeon inserted a drain for a few days until it resolved. It's amazing to me that she has hair growing on the left side of her head because that flap of skin was laid open a couple of times. I told the doctor jokingly at one point, "If you open that up one more time, can you just put a zipper in?"

One of the other specialists that we added to Paula's team in Ohio was a rehabilitative ophthalmologist. I had no idea that such a thing existed, but it became another specialist that we needed to know about.

Paula's eyes were not lined up well with one another, so she had double vision. Her right eye didn't track correctly because the muscles that control it weren't fully reconnected or working well yet. We went to the rehabilitative ophthalmologist and she made her a set of glasses with a prism built into the right lens. This prism shifted what Paula was seeing through that eye a degree or two toward the center line of her face. If you have a stroke survivor or a head injury patient that is complaining of double vision, I recommend consulting with a rehabilitative ophthalmologist if there are any indications of a problem.

Dr. Drusilla Grant was neat. She taught rehabilitative ophthalmology in colleges around the country as a visiting lecturer. Luckily, she was practicing in Akron so we could see her locally. She applied treatments such as light therapy that improved parts of the cognitive processes. She assessed Paula and told her to stare at blue-green light for a little while every day. The color cyan was beneficial for her. It helped to reconnect and activate some parts of her brain that weren't working well yet. It feels touchy-feely in nature, but Dr. Grant used both the scientific process and her intuition to assign exercises.

Dr. Grant did another test on Paula. They have you put your chin on what looks like a small planetarium turned ninety degrees so the cone of it is parallel to the floor and you're focused on the center of the hemisphere. You stare into the hemisphere and they show random Xs on this planetarium. When you see an X, you push a button that you're holding in your hand. The sphere goes all the way around to the top, bottom, and sides of your face and tests your peripheral vision. The first time Paula did that test, she saw none of the Xs on the right side of her nose. She had no field of vision there.

The doctor gave me a detailed description of how the eyes and brain work together. Part of the visual inputs of one eye goes to the left side of the brain and also to the right, and part of the other eye goes another way. They get mixed together in the brain to make up what we see. My head exploded when she described it to me and I said, "Do what you gotta do and we'll be back next week." Even with all the brain training she performed, to this day, Paula doesn't see things very well on the right side.

I don't see them consistently, but sometimes I can see.

Paula has some peripheral vision on the right side now, but it's not nearly as good as it is on the left side. I guess it involves that cross-sided interconnection. She can't see and recognize many things on the right side, but she can see a few things sometimes. The brain is very complex. She can see some movement, but in many cases, she can't see an object that's not moving.

The doctors and therapists described another thing to me called neglect. When a person who has suffered a head injury has a weak side, they neglect it. Paula couldn't move her whole right side for almost a year, so she neglected it and it became weaker as a result. I always thought that you neglect it because it wasn't useful, and only recently one of her therapists told me that you neglect it because your brain really doesn't recognize that it exists. It's not a conscious decision to neglect parts of your body.

This therapist also described what another patient experienced. He held the patient's hand and rubbed it, but she didn't know it was her hand from which she was feeling sensations. That was an example of severe neglect in a stroke survivor. There's another term that the doctors use called disuse. That's when something is ignored because it's not useful. I don't know how to figure out where Paula is on that continuum. We don't have to classify exactly where Paula is, though. We just have to keep working on her using her right arm and hand as much as she can.

There is a certain therapy where your strong hand is actually tied up so that you can't use it and you have to use your weak hand for all the exercises. Paula tries to use her right hand more and more. She's using it to help put toothpaste on her toothbrush, turn the water on and off, and cut vegetables for her salad.

We had an occupational therapist that looked at my shoulder and said, "Your shoulder is totally screwed up and separated." He said there was nothing I could do but to "get it welded" together. We went to see someone and the guy there didn't look like a doctor at all. I said, "Who are you?" He said, "I'm your doctor," and I said, "You don't look like a doctor!" I asked him, "Do you know anyone who can work with a shoulder? I've been told that my shoulder is totally screwed up and I should just have it put together." He told me to come in and they did an x-ray. He told me, "Your shoulder is not totally screwed up; you just need to work it."

Over time, through disuse of parts of your body, the muscles atrophy and weird things happen. The worst of these for Paula was osteopenia and osteoporosis. She was post-menopausal when she had the accident, so osteoporosis and osteopenia - bone weakness and bone thinness - were both concerns but she only developed them after the accident. Using your body and engaging in weight-bearing exercises both build bone mass, but Paula wasn't bearing weight, so she developed osteopenia. She took Fosamax and some other drugs to help build up her bone mass.

Her shoulder issue developed because she wasn't using her right arm, so the ligaments and muscles in her shoulder weakened and stretched as gravity took control. Her stride was such that when she stepped out with her right foot, it jerked her right arm down, so we started working more on her gait. It wasn't separated because that would mean the shoulder was out of joint, but the joint isn't quite as tight as it should be.

I had gotten to where in the scooter I'd roll around the whole block, and so I was rolling along and thought, I can straighten my arm because I was doing this thing. I thought I could do it, but unfortunately I didn't know to watch the shoulders. Both too much and too little movement is detrimental, but it's the underlying disuse of a body part that's really bad.

I thought I'd keep it up. Through that, I lost a lot of use of my hand because I used to be able to move my thumb and my finger.

We were ignorant because her hand wasn't useful, so unless she was actually doing therapy with it, she would ignore her hand.

I think I used it for a lot of stuff that I would do. When I was cleaning the barn and stuff like that, I didn't have my hand tucked up. I had it doing stuff for a while.

With a brain injury, whether it's minor or severe, all those systems in your brain are affected in some way. Paula's were dramatically affected. Every little indication, like the double vision and the arm, were symptoms or indicators of a body system staying the same, getting better, or having a problem - all at their own pace.

The challenge is that there's a specialist out there for darn near every issue you can imagine. We've had to deal with odd things you'd never expect to deal with, like Paula's toenails on her right foot growing differently. The nail on her big toe gets thick and has to be thinned and trimmed with a Dremel tool because you can't cut it. Sometimes we have to go to a podiatrist (foot doctor) so he can numb her toe and cut her toenail way back.

# Chapter 16

# Gaining Independence

When Paula came home from HealthSouth, we still had the horses that we were riding in the accident. They were out in the barn and I was still taking care of them. I would ask her about it occasionally, but she would never express any interest in going out and seeing the horses. This was amazing because she lived and breathed horses before her accident.

I don't really know why that is, and she doesn't really remember why she didn't want to go see them. Was it fear? Was it just that she didn't know what they were for? I don't know how other people would deal with this. I've never talked to anybody in support groups that we went to about this.

Sometime after I got over my broken hip, we got an electric wheelchair that my mother-in-law had used before she died. I used it inside the house and could use it outside a little, too. It would get stuck in the driveway and in the grass sometimes. We didn't have the small four-wheel outdoor scooter that I have now.

I was doing laundry one day and I heard the dogs barking. I thought it was UPS or something and I roll and look out the door. There were two horses in our driveway talking to my two horses.

There were no people, so I said, "Oh shit," got in my electric wheelchair, told the dogs to stay there, and went down the gravel driveway in the wheelchair. The horses weren't there, so I'm rolling around and a guy rides by on a bicycle, so I said, "Hey! Where are those horses?" He told me, "In your backyard!" and I saw that the horses had come down our driveway. We had a field and a long driveway and nice grass. The guy came over and asked, "What do you want me to do for them?"

I told him, "It would really be nice if we could put them in the field beside our horses." He asked me how we would do that, and I said, "We could open this gate and you just have to stand there to keep them from running through." I went over to the horses in my wheelchair and told them, "It's okay, it's okay." I led one of the horses and drove the scooter.

I told the biker what he needed to do. I couldn't try to put the horses in the field because it had rained and the land was soggy. "Get the horse and take it to the tree and tie it up." He did that and came back and I said, "Can you hold the gate again?" He held the gate and I went over and got one of the horses and said, "Shhh. Come on."

As we were moving, the horse sort of spooked and I told him to quiet down. The horses weren't afraid of me. I petted him and brought him up to the gate. The biker and I got both the horses in and shut the gate. He said, "What now?" and I told him, "It would be good if you could take the bridles off because they can get caught. You don't need to fool with the saddle, just take the bridle off." And he did. Then he untied the other horse and got his bridle off. He asked me what he should do with the bridles and I told him to bring them over to me and to call Doug.

I think she wanted to show off about what she had done. It was pretty neat that she could calm and lead the horses from her electric wheelchair.

We called Doug and the police and told them there were two

horses here. The police said they would send someone out. A van went by slowly and then stopped, backed up, and came down our road. There was a lady driving the car and two girls in the back. The girls did not know the lady; they were just walking down the road and had hitched a ride to go look for their horses. They told the lady that they saw which direction their horses went and said, "Hey, can you take us this way?"

So they came in and saw their horses and said, "Ahhh, thank you!" and gave us both hugs and took the horses. Everything was okay. They brought their horses up and thanked us again. The lady in the van who had dropped the girls off left. I thought about how cool that was. The biker guy told me, "That was really nice. I didn't know anything about horses, and next week I'm going down to the Kentucky Derby horse race." I showed him Clypso and Boogie and told him, "They're saddlebreds."

I gave him a short horse lesson and thanked him for his help before he got on his bicycle and left. I didn't know any of them—not the girls or the driver or the biker. After all that, I went back and I emailed Guilene, a good friend who is very horsey person, saying, "This is great!" and telling her how cool it was that everything had happened like that. They had left one of the reins, a long leather lead line, there. We got in the car and tried to find where the horses and the girls were and we could never find them. They had been riding for miles.

Anytime we saw anybody and Doug told them that I fell off a horse, I would say, "It wasn't the horse's fault." Whether I spoke well or not, "It wasn't the horse's fault" was always easy for me to say.

It almost never is their fault, and that's why it's called an accident (and why it's the title of this book).

One day more than a year after she came home, Paula said, "I want to go out and see the horses." I never really attached a lot of significance to getting her to go out to the barn again. She never was able to talk about why she hadn't wanted to go out to the barn up to that point. In the same way, someone who fell down a flight of stairs might be afraid of those stairs.

I didn't know how to build that into our process of getting on and driving to recover. It didn't feel right to force her to go out to the barn. We just let her choose her tasks at her own pace. When she finally did go out to the barn, it didn't seem like a big deal to either one of us. Paula just went out there one day, said hello to her friends, and started cleaning up the feed and tack room.

# CHAPTER 17

# BACK IN THE SADDLE AGAIN

Boogie was four when we got him and eight when I fell. About two years after my accident, he got very ill. The vet said he had a bad problem. A lot of horses have colic and die from that, but Boogie had come down with something and his body was in bad shape. We had to have him put to sleep. He was only nine years old. We said goodbye and then buried him in the back pasture.

Clypso took off running to the end of the field. He had not run for a long time. We had two fields and we opened the gate and Clypso ran to the end of the field, and then walked back. We thought he was just running along the fence line as Boogie's spirit galloped off to greener pastures. Clypso died two or three years after that. He colicked (twisted piece of intestine) and couldn't be saved. I went over to him and thought, "There ain't nothing we can do about it."

It turned out that Boogie had developed something called equine metabolic disorder, something very similar to Type 2 Diabetes in humans. In horses, it causes them to founder, a condition where the structure of the foot changes such that they can't put any pressure on the foot without it causing unbearable pain. Boogie foundered in all four feet within a week and a half, so there was nothing that could reasonably be done to save him. It was a very sad day on many levels when we had to have him put down.

When Paula had been home for a while after breaking her hip, she got stronger. She started to ask about riding again. We started looking into therapeutic horseback riding. Friends of mine thought I was crazy. They said, "How can you let her get back on a horse?" I said, "How can I not?"

Horses were and are such an important part of her and her life.

We identified a really good local riding center about twelve miles from our house. It's highly regarded in Hartville, Ohio and around the country. I went over to meet with the people there and explained who I was and Paula's situation. I told them I wanted to get her on a horse, and soon. The staff told me it was a long process. They said that I'd have to get doctor's waivers and have us evaluated and that it could take five or six months. I went home thinking that it wasn't going to work. But four weeks later out of sheer determination, Paula started her first lesson.

We saw the benefits of therapeutic riding; it's a wonderful thing for people with strokes and head injuries, and is good for a lot of people. Particularly those with head injuries where gait is involved. The walking motion of the horse increases the body's core strength and balance. It is very helpful in activating and strengthening the large and small muscles in your stomach and back that let you sit up straight, hold your head up, balance yourself, and have better peripheral vision and coordination.

The therapist told us that the horse replicates the human

gait and the walking pattern better than any machine, other than a treadmill. If you watch somebody walking and watch somebody going by on a horse, their upper body is doing pretty much the same thing. In Paula's case, the emotional benefit was also amazing. Horses and people can have a really special connection and emotional bond.

When Paula got back up on a horse, we saw amazing things, both with her and with others in the program. When she started, she could not move her right hand and didn't use it, but when we got her up in the saddle, I put the reins in her hand and after about two weeks she started using it to hold the reins. When she'd get off the horse and into the car, her right hand didn't work anymore. She must have been accessing different parts of the brain. Some would call it muscle memory, but I think it was deep brain memories in different parts of the brain.

Paula rode for a little over two years. Unfortunately, there was a weight limit of two hundred pounds and when she creeped over that a little bit, they made her stop riding. That was a great loss for Paula, because it had helped her with her gait and leg strength so much since she was holding on with her legs. Furthermore, it was a great emotional benefit for her to be back on a horse again.

There was a lady who started riding with Paula who had multiple sclerosis (MS). The first night she came, two of us had to literally lift her out of the wheelchair and put her on the horse. Three months and only twelve riding sessions later, she was coming in and out with a walker because it had rebuilt her core strength and balance so much. She is still riding to this day.

My first exposure to therapeutic riding was serving as

Paula's side walker. I went to the volunteer training and told them, "If she's going to fall off another horse, she's gonna fall on me. I'm not going to leave this up to somebody else." I was her personal side walker. She needed two of us initially, as they worked her through an individualized plan of progress.

The goal for Paula was to build strength and be able to ride more independently eventually. Early on, we had to hold Paula up because she didn't have the strength and balance to stay on the horse. After a few weeks, we didn't have to hold on as much. We just held the saddle and remained next to her just in case she teetered. She continued to gain strength and improve her balance. About eight months later, one of the side walkers went away. Shortly after that I could walk farther from the horse and not have contact. She did still need a horse leader though, who helped by leading the horse on a rope and making sure that the horse didn't spook.

Later in the second year, Paula started riding more or less independently. The horse leader was eight feet away, just barely holding onto the rope and Paula was actually steering the horse. Cognitively, that's important because Paula had to take in a lot of sensory inputs, including instructions and cues from the instructor saying to turn left or right as well as what was going on with other riders in the ring at the same time.

They had Paula do things in the ring like picking brightly colored rings off the right colored peg and putting them on the other peg while she was riding by. She had to deliver mail to a mailbox. She had to take stuffed animals off one post and put them in a bucket on the other side of the ring. She had to ride patterns around the ring and go from one specific spot in the ring to another. And so on. It was a very powerful thing to observe.

But I wasn't very good at being nice and sincere.

Paula gave the instructor a lot of grief because she acted up a bit in classes, but in a fun way. She rode in an adult class during the evening one night a week. There were three or four people in her class, a couple of people with MS, another stroke survivor, and Paula. There were issues because Paula had contracture, muscle stiffness in her right leg which caused her toes to drop and her calf muscle and Achilles tendon to tighten, so she was putting a lot of pressure on her feet.

She ended up almost wearing through the skin on the little bone on the base of her little toe on her right foot because she was putting so much pressure on it by not only horseback riding, but just through everyday walking. That became a real issue when we couldn't bend Paula's foot to a ninety-degree angle, which is important for walking. We learned that we had to have her Achilles tendon lengthened under anesthesia with an Achilles tenotomy.

We had another great doctor who performed the surgery, which entailed making little incisions in Paula's Achilles tendon to cut halfway through it in several places and then stretching it out and putting her in a cast. It healed and grew back longer. She then had more range of motion in her foot. That's another one of those routine procedures that I was exposed to. It was not a matter of survival, it was a matter of what we can do to help Paula be in a position to get better and regain as much normalcy as possible.

No matter who you are or where you live, there's a therapeutic riding center near you. In North America alone, there are more than 850 centers affiliated with PATH International, the Professional Association of Therapeutic Horsemanship. Some large cities have two or three centers.

The PATH International website (www.path-intl.org) has a locator so you can find one near you. I encourage you to explore this as part of the recovery process whether your loved one liked horses or not, but particularly if they did. Head injuries that girls and women suffer from are more often than not from horseback riding accidents, according to Paula's neurosurgeon. Among young men, it's mostly automobile or motorcycle accidents.

Therapeutic riding is good for a lot of things, but particularly head injuries. Aquatic therapy was another great exercise for helping to improve walking. We participated in aquatic therapy in both Ohio and in North Carolina. It was a great way to work on improving the gait without the risk of falling. The resistance offered by the water as you walk along in chest-deep water is also good for strengthening all the muscles involved in walking. It also helped her improve her sense of balance.

One of our biggest fears has been, and continues to be, falls. Paula's balance still isn't good. Her gait is not normalized and we continue to work on that with therapy, but she has fallen a number of times. She hasn't fallen as much recently, which is good because when she fell in the first few years after the accident, she suffered compression fractures in her spine.

As a result, she's lost about two inches of height. I don't care about the height; what I care about are the little tiny fractures and the curvature in her spine. She has developed scoliosis both from the muscle weakness and from some of the compression fractures.

In Ohio, I got to where I could stand up and do stuff. Going down the hallway to get to the garage, I opened the door and was starting to fall over, so I stopped myself. I put a hole in the wall, but I stopped myself. I've heard from people that tell me, "You've just gotten so much better!"and I think, "I wasn't that bad!" but apparently I'm better. I don't know what has changed.

I would go up to my friend, Jackson's, and he would be in his tractor pulling out some posts and I'd ask if I could sit there and watch him. He was an older farmer and someone I could talk to. I'd roll over with the dogs and I could let our dogs loose in his yard, and the dogs were really cool and would stay around me.

He lived about a quarter mile or a half-mile away when I used to roll down to see him. I'd go in my scooter. The house where we lived used to be an old corn field and somebody bought the land, so now it was houses, and then some space and another house, and then Jackson. He had fifty acres. He had some land that he rented out to another farmer and a tractor trail that went back to the woods past the open land.

I was always looking for something to do. In the early days, I would go up to Jackson's. But one time I went up to Jackson's and there were two cars, and I said, I don't want to be a bother, so I went around. There was a nice yard but he had a pipe from his house going down into the ground. There was a little ditch where the pipe ran that I didn't see. So, my scooter tipped over and I fell on my side.

I yelled, "Damn. Jackson!" and he came over and said, "What are you doing?" I told him, "Well, it was a nice day. I thought I would just lay here and enjoy it." He was about eighty or eighty-one, a young guy, and he asked, "Anything I can do?" and I said, "Can you get my scooter up?" It was on its side and he came and picked it up, and I said, "Can you help me get up?" and he told me, "I don't know."

I had never noticed that he was short. I put my hands on his shoulders and they were too short, and I told him, "Nah. I don't want you to get hurt," so I called Doug. At the time, we were getting a new roof and I asked Doug to come over. He came zooming over and got me up, asking if I was okay and I told him I was. Then Doug went back, but I just stayed.

Jackson was fun to talk to because he didn't give me the, "Oh, you poor creature." I met a lot of people that asked, "What did you do?" and I'd tell them and say, "You wanna feel my head?" Ninety percent of people would say, "Wow, you've got a lot of bumps on your head," and I would agree. I'm trying to get better. I see people who complain about their legs hurting and I say, "Well, enjoy them." You can end up like that. I'd see kids and go, "Do me a favor. Go out and play for me, because I can't do that anymore, so enjoy what you're doing." If I see any horsey people, I say, "Do me a favor. Tell the horse 'thank you'."

# Part Three:

# Thrive

Thrive (thrahyv) : a verb meaning to grow or develop successfully, or to flourish or succeed.

*"It takes but one positive thought when given a chance to survive and thrive to overpower an entire army of negative thoughts."*
—Robert H. Schuller

We've all heard the expression, "When life gives you lemons, make lemonade." When I retired from the navy, our plan was for me to find a job teaching business classes at a small college somewhere. Mount Union College and I seemed to be a perfect match. I wanted to do exactly what they hired me to do. I was loving it and, by all accounts, doing a pretty good job too. Since we had my navy retired pay and good health insurance from the navy, too, we planned on spending a good deal of my teaching salary on airplane tickets and hotel rooms in far off places during the summers. Paula's accident, a little more than two years into this new chapter in our lives put those plans on indefinite hold.

Instead, we found out that Paula could get in and out of a motor home with my assistance, so we started to look at different options to see if there was a floor plan that we liked. We needed one that would be safe enough for Paula to get around in and do things in relative safety.

On her birthday in 2005, we found the right one. It was a thirty-seven foot long, 1998 Fleetwood Discovery that had a little over 15,000 miles on it; barely broken in for a diesel engine. We bought it and outfitted it with dishes, linens, and all the other stuff you need to live for two to three months at a time. I installed the running gear on my PT Cruiser that would allow me to tow it. We figured out how to fit Paula's four-wheel outdoor mobility scooter in one of the storage lockers on the bottom of "the rig," as we called it.

I don't know who said, "In the end, the quality of your life depends largely on how well you deal with plan B," but I learned to deeply respect that wisdom during my career in the navy and afterwards. Our plan B became doing some travelling around the country in our motor home and enjoying some of the beautiful places and friendly people that make it so special. I actually might have preferred to live in the motor home full time but Paula really likes the idea of having a mailbox. As a result, our plan B also included my leaving Mount Union College and moving somewhere new to build our *forever home*.

For our entire married life up to this point, we had moved somewhere to work there. This was a very different experience, as we were searching for someplace that we wanted to live, and thrive.

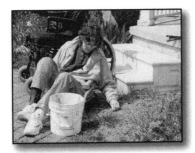

Paula Weeding again - not going as
fast, but loving it nonetheless

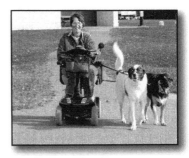

Paula's new mobility scooter
opened up new horizons for her,
and the dogs

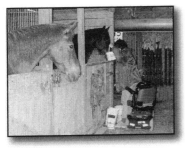

Paula feeding Clypso(l) &
Boogie (r). Paula was riding Boogie
& Doug was riding Clypso the day
of her accident

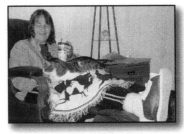

Paula recovering from surgery to
lengthen her Achilles tendon

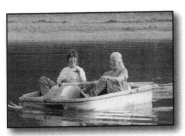

Paula & a friend having fun in
New Jersey on one of our trips

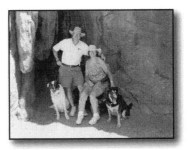

The "family" at Garden of the Gods
in Colorado on one of our trips

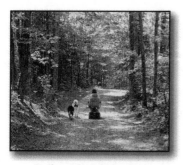

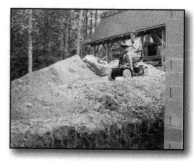

Paula exploring the new neighborhood in North Carolina. She loves the trees

Paula supervising construction of our new Home in North Carolina

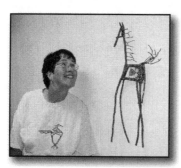

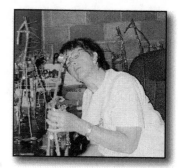

Paula admiring Waldo, one of her beautiful Untamed Horses, 2012

Paula creating one of her beautiful Untamed Horses, 2013

# CHAPTER 18

# BURNING OUT & MOVING ON

Paula came home in August of 2002 and I taught full time at Mount Union College until 2009. Our pace of life was getting to be more than I could handle. By the end of the school year in 2005, it was clear to me that I was at a great risk of burning out. I was burning my candle at both ends and some in the middle. I also needed to try to do some things for myself. For instance, I didn't play golf for more than five years after Paula's injury. I used to play two or three days a week when I was in the navy. It's a form of stress management for me and I just didn't have the time to enjoy it any longer. At school, I didn't feel like I was able to give the students everything they deserved, and I wasn't going to shortchange them.

At the end of the 2005 school year, I figured that we were in a position where we could fully retire. We started actively thinking about where we would like to retire to and build or buy our forever home.

During the Christmas break in 2005, we visited some friends who were moving from Charlotte to Etowah, North Carolina, which is near Brevard. We rented a cabin in nearby Mills River and had a great visit with our friends.

While there, we also connected with a realtor who showed us some land in Henderson County.

We drove down to Brevard and liked how the town felt. It was a small, very welcoming town. We stopped to eat lunch in *Rocky's Soda Shop* while we were there. Halfway through lunch, I looked across the table and said to Paula, "I feel like I've lived here for forty years." She agreed. This is saying a lot for a couple who had moved every two to three years for the majority of their married life. After a little more research about quality of life and real estate prices, Brevard rose to the top of our list of serious candidates for places for us to move to and start thriving.

We decided to move to Brevard. My mom lived in West Asheville, about thirty miles north of there, for more than twenty years before she died. I'd visit her and she'd show me places she enjoyed. We had looked around in this area and it felt good. We talked to a realtor in Hendersonville and looked at some land, but Hendersonville was too big and just didn't feel right to me.

One day we drove down this road and pulled up to where this land was for sale, and I said, "This is it." This feels good. I want to be in the mountains and I want trees. We don't have a view here, but we have trees. I am truly addicted to trees. I didn't like the place that we bought in Ohio because it had no trees around the house. I kept saying, "I don't like this house, I don't like this house." The land we found in Brevard was just what I was looking for.

Paula grew up mostly in the Blue Ridge Mountains of the Shenandoah Valley in Virginia. I grew up in Pittsburgh which is also very mountainous. I spent a lot of my summers and weekends with my father at a Boy Scout camp in the Laurel Mountains of western Pennsylvania, which is part of the Appalachian Mountains as well. So, we really wanted to live in a mountainous region. The mountains that we saw out west in Colorado and New Mexico were too big and too rough for us. We both like mountains and the North Carolina area. We were very interested in living somewhere in the triangle formed by Johnson City, Tennessee; Franklin, North Carolina; and Tryon, North Carolina because of the climate, weather, and culture. Also, North Carolina (along with several other states) doesn't tax retired military pay.

It was on my birthday that we went and looked at motor homes and I was so excited. Doug found one and said, "I want you to come and look at it." Motor homes have several steps, but this one seemed easy for me to get into and out of. We went in and looked at the whole inside before sitting on the couch, visualizing actually living in it. We sat there for about thirty minutes, just getting the feel of the place.

I told Doug this was it. It was an older one, but that didn't matter. We brought it home. Doug drove the motor home in, parked it, and asked me, "Do you want to take the dogs for a drive in the new rig?" I said yes.

The dogs and I got in and we went around and realized motor homes don't turn like a car, they have a long end and you have to watch the entire side very carefully when you make turns, just like a big bus or truck. The driveway was straight but Doug had made a loop in it. He drove it around the loop and we went "bonk" on something! I told Doug that the dogs and I were going to get out. It turned out that Doug had found a large boulder we had in the planter. It messed up about ten feet of the passenger side of the motor home. It ruined two of the storage compartment doors and bent the frame for those compartments, too. But he straightened it out and replaced the doors. Soon after that, we got ready to go meet some friends for our first long distance camping trip in the motor home.

We met them in a state park in southern West Virginia; that was the first camping that we had done and it was just so cool. I liked just being out and talking to people and not being in Ohio. Doug would unhook the car, pull into a camping space, and get my scooter out of the basement storage bin. I'd get on it, take the dogs, and leave. Doug would finish setting everything up and getting it ready to live in because I had no idea how to handle that stuff.

I would roll around and talk to people, and the next day when Doug and I would both walk around, people would say, "Hi Paula!" I would talk to anybody. Walking around, we met new people and that was cool. We spent time outside without the computer and the cell phone. And the dogs liked it.

We went to New River–it starts in Virginia but goes through the mountains of West Virginia. There was a long path that you could see the river from; we didn't bring my scooter, so I got to walk all the way out with Doug's help. It was just so cool. I wasn't able to play in the river. Doug and I later went camping by ourselves somewhere. This trip served to be proof that we could do it and enjoy it a lot, too.

Later we went to southern New Jersey to see where we once lived and visit with friends who still lived there. It was cool to see where we'd lived and see our friends again. Coming back, we visited the last roommate that I had in Monroeville. After that, we went home and then took off to go out west. It was really cool to just see the west and all the different things out there. That was our thirtieth anniversary.

In 2006, we loaded up the motor home and headed west to see Paula's sister in New Mexico. First we drove from Ohio to Illinois to visit my cousin. Then, we went to Denver to visit some friends from Guam—Ginny, the friend who came to Ohio to help out when Paula first came home. From Denver, we headed south to New Mexico to spend time with Paula's sister.

From there, we headed to Brevard to look at land. We ended up buying 2.5 acres of land just south of town on top of Becky Mountain at an elevation of three thousand feet. It was the beginning of our plan to retire and move south. We put in the offer to buy the land on our thirtieth anniversary and it was accepted. This was our thirtieth anniversary, one of those speed limit anniversaries that end in a zero or a five, so it was destined to be. It was sort of an anniversary present to each other. That was also the date of Paula's last seizure, which was serendipitous. We continue to celebrate both.

Not far from our new home site there is a nice little campground co-located with a horse farm where people board and ride horses. It was a perfect place to park the motor home over the next few summers (and even some of our Thanksgiving and Christmas breaks) as we got the land ready to build on and build a barn to park the motor home in while we worked on the house.

At three thousand feet on top of a mountain, if you don't have water, you don't build, so the next summer (2007), we went back down to Brevard to drill the well and bring in all the utilities: electric, phone, cable TV. We also flattened off a spot for a large barn for the motor home. I ran sewer, water, and electric out to the barn location. Paula worked on clearing small trees and clearing the weeds off several parts of the land.

The following summer, in 2008, we built the barn. I dug some big, round holes and poured concrete for the sixteen 6x6 posts that would hold up the roof. This is a pretty big barn: 26x48 feet.

We built the rough structure and on our anniversary that year, backed the motor home in, plugged in, and lived on our own property while continuing to work on the barn. The trusses and roof weren't in place yet, but we really wanted to have the motor home up there and be self-sufficient on our anniversary before heading back to Ohio.

Paula couldn't help much with the actual construction, so

she worked the land a bit, cutting down some small trees, making herself some trails down through the wooded parts of the land, and introducing herself to the neighbors.

Our plan for moving to North Carolina was to live in the motor home on our property while we built the house. I'd be the general contractor and manage the schedule, order the materials, hire the contractors, and work with them on the actual construction and finishing of the house.

We went home that fall and put our 11.5 acre hobby farm on the market. I gave my notice at the college, which I hated to do because it was a dream job in many ways. I knew that I couldn't keep doing it in the way that I knew it should be done, so it was time to leave.

We all know what happened in 2008: The financial world in general and the housing market in particular fell apart. There we were, putting our place in northeast Ohio on the market, which was one of the *ground zeros* of the national housing market collapse.

I didn't listen to my own advice that horse properties are different–they sell–so I got nervous and I asked Mount Union if I could stay another year. They were happy to have me, so I signed on to do it, but then we sold the house a month and a half later, without even using a seller's agent. Did I mention that horse properties are special and don't follow the same rules as other types of real estate?

Because of my commitment to stay another year, we had to go out and find an apartment to rent. We found a one-bedroom place that was built with accessibility in mind and was less than a mile from my office.

Paula absolutely hated this apartment because it was a small place with no trees and she didn't have her own yard. But she could take the dogs for long walks through the community in her scooter, and it was close enough that she would come over to campus and visit.

As I mentioned earlier, our plan was to spend a good deal of my college salary on airplane tickets and hotel rooms going to see places that we'd been before (Bali, Japan, and Thailand) and even some new places during the summers. Of course, the accident changed all that. Flying was not something we could really think about doing, although the doctors have now cleared her to fly. The logistics of flying, mobility, and having a scooter on the other end just seemed too much to try to coordinate. In addition, the doctors didn't particularly recommend that Paula fly during the first several years of her recovery because of the pressure changes that you can experience in an airplane. Her brain might not take those well for a while.

My doctor only recently told me that I can go on an airplane, but I haven't tried it yet. The motor home allows us to travel. When I was *normal*, I would take my horse riding and work on the farm. I wasn't that sociable. I would go out and see people, but only for ten minutes or so, and then I would go on. But when I got to where I couldn't go riding, I would talk to people for longer because it was something to do.

While we were living in the motor home on our property while building the house, we had an ice storm that broke off many of the tops of the trees. I found out that the tulip poplar trees had little spikes at the tip of the branches that were left from the seed pods after the seeds had all flown away. I thought they were pretty and wondered what I could make with them.

Later, when the electricians were working on wiring the house, they'd leave wire pieces lying around and I'd collect them. I would keep them in a five-gallon bucket so that we could take it and recycle it. I had a small pile of wire when all the treetops came down and there were a lot of broken pieces of treetops lying around. I wondered if I could make a horse out of the sticks and wires, so I made one.

It wasn't a very good horse, but Doug and others who saw it thought it was very nice. I decided I could do better, so I made another one that was better. I also made some wreathes out of grapevines, but I wouldn't do that again. I started making the horses a while after we moved in the house. I could cut the wood up and make some horses, but I couldn't do the wire because I couldn't tighten it enough. I had done some of it, but it was still too wobbly, so I got Doug to finish the wire. It drove me crazy having to wait for him to do that.

# CHAPTER 19

# DESIGNING & BUILDING OUR FOREVER HOME

Up till now, we hadn't actually finished designing the house we were going to build on our land. We still weren't sure we could build one, as we didn't know for sure if we could find water when we dug a well. We spent one summer on our new land just running in the utilities and having the well dug.

When it was time to drill the well, we hired a "witcher." Some people call them dowsers, but a lot of people call them witchers in North Carolina. She came out and used her forked stick and special skills to recommend a good place to find water. I'm a pretty rational, scientific guy, but I believe in this for some reason. I'm convinced that some people are just wired differently and can find water, and she did. I don't know if there would've been water anywhere else we drilled, but I do know a guy right down the hill who spent a lot of money drilling three dry holes in the ground. He didn't hire a witcher.

While we were watching the workers bring in the utilities and dig the well, I had a lot of time to reflect on what life would be like on top of this mountain. We had talked some about this before buying the land, but being here and turning it into an actual home site made it much more real. Because of the fact that Paula's world would shrink, I was very worried about moving to the top of this mountain. We knew that we would both love this area, the scenery, and the people. She'd be able to meet lots of different people. Where we lived in Ohio, she could get on her scooter and ride for miles safely if she wanted to, on straight, rural farm roads. You could see what was coming for miles. She could roll along for miles, but couldn't talk to many neighbors (most of them worked) or go to any areas with lots of trees. She really wasn't as brave there as she would later become in North Carolina.

In North Carolina, her world got much smaller in many ways. When we moved to this new place, the roads are a little bit more dangerous. The places she can go are more limited. It's also gotten larger recently because we have a larger circle of mutual friends now.

Typically, when a married couple is working, they each their own circles of friends at their work and they're not always very involved with each other's friends. That was the case in Ohio. I had a lot of friends and colleagues at work that Paula didn't interact with, and she had friends that I didn't interact with.

I'd spend my time rolling around the neighborhood in my scooter. When we'd parked the motor home and were building the house, I would go on long distance rolls to the end of the road. Aik Teong came to see us one year and we went for a long roll in my outdoor scooter. OK, I rolled and he walked. He and I went around a whole subdivision nearby, and I thought, "Cool. I've never done that before!" I've done a few more long roads, and I made some paths down through our woods.

I also drew a lot of pictures on the computer. I did the exercises that the physical therapists had given me. It's important to keep working to improve on what already works and to try to get new things working, too.

I'm just not good at sitting and not doing something. I don't spend much time in the garden anymore, because I can't get in to do the things I want to do.

When we talked about this before we moved down here, I said, "Paula, we bought that land, but your world is going to be smaller there because you are not going to be able to drive your scooter down into town."

We do put her scooter on the car and go to the farmer's market, the nearby state and national forests, the Biltmore Estate, and street festivals in Brevard. She likes leaving me behind and taking off to see people and the places we go. At the festivals, she goes and talks to nearly all the vendors in their booths and a lot of the people on the street. At the farmer's market, she'll take off in one direction with one dog and I go the other way with the other dog. If we go to Biltmore and she wants to go look at something, I say, "Go ahead. We'll hook back up in a little while." But we have to go somewhere first before she has that freedom.

Doug was talking about maybe getting a house in town and I said, "I can't roll around on that area because it's small and I don't have any ability to move around." Town doesn't suit me as well as being up here on the mountain.

I wouldn't want to live in town; I like it up here. In some ways, Paula's world up here is like a big fish in a small pond. She's a fixture on the mountain now, so people actually stop their cars when she's out there to stop and talk.

We designed the house that we built; or rather, Paula designed the house we built. We knew what the land was like, the slope and which way south was, so we could take advantage of the winter sunlight. I would bring home books from the library and CDs from Lowe's and download floor plans on the internet.

We went out to all the model home shows and many open houses to see what we liked and didn't like. I'd show Paula a floor plan and she'd say, "No, I don't like that." After about three weeks of that I said, "Okay, you don't get to say that anymore. For every plan I show you, you've got to tell me two or three things you like about it and two or three things you don't like about it."

I started keeping a list of what she liked and didn't like, because she wasn't very good at telling me why she did or didn't like it. I had to force that issue. One night about six months later, using a cheap piece of software, I scratched together a floor plan based on our conversations of what we'd seen and liked and her list of things she liked and didn't like.

I printed it out and brought that floor plan down in the morning. Paula looked at it and said, "That's it, where did you get that?" I said, "Well, you designed it." We had a year to finalize the house design and go to home shows to look at cabinets we liked and all the other things you have to decide upon when building a house.

In May of 2009, we packed everything that hadn't already been sent to North Carolina into the motor home, drove to our mountain home site, and backed the motor home into the barn on our property. We plugged it in to high speed internet, cable TV, telephone, and full hookups. It was time to build our forever home and get on with the business of thriving in our new hometown. We had arrived!

We had taken out one sofa in the motor home and replaced it with a table for my computer. If I had to get stuck inside for any reason, I could work on the computer. I could watch what was going on outside, too. At night, when we were in the motor home, I played games on the computer, used the computer, or drew because I'm not good at sitting and reading. Even when I was normal, I would read only at nighttime. I wasn't going out and sitting on the porch and reading—I just wanted to do something.

We set the motor home up as a place for the family (Paula, me, our dog, and our cat) to live. It was also my construction office, because I did the general contracting. Most of my career in the navy was spent in contracting, logistics, and program management; so I figured if I couldn't run the construction of my own house, I ought to give some of my retired pay back.

We did learn some interesting twists, such as when you're building a house you first settle on the framing crew and then find out which contractors they like for the follow-on work. Sourcing contractors is important. My background in contracting and contract management helped a lot. It also worked in our favor that we were building at the very bottom of the housing construction cycle in 2009, because the contractors didn't have much work and were readily available to work with us.

We had one set of contractors come to give us a quote one day. One of them drove back the next day and undercut his own quote. He told me, "I really want this job, and I'm gonna do it for this." In that particular case, I said, "Nah, you can have it for your original bid."

We did some interesting things to find contractors; we

went to the local greasy spoon restaurant where contractors would go to eat breakfast and lunch. We'd watch how they treated the waiters and waitresses. If they were nice to them, we thought they were probably a good person and we'd have them up to give us a quote. It was a good application of the old philosophy that, "Somebody who's not nice to the waitress is not a nice person."

We lived in the motor home for about a year while we built the place. It was hard work, but fun: I worked with all the crews, I ordered all the material, helped cut wood, helped set the trusses, helped unload trucks, and managed the building of our forever home.

We did go through a lot of fits and foibles involving the long-term routine of adapting to our *new normal* during this period.

For instance, Paula was on three different anti-seizure drugs. I take a few medications myself and we both take some vitamins and supplements. So, every two weeks I pack two pill containers with four compartments for each day of the week to hold all our pills for the next two weeks. It helps to have that routine to follow.

I once got her Phenobarbital and my Flecainide mixed up. The ramifications of that were interesting: Phenobarbital is a tranquilizer and anti-seizure medication, and Flecainide is what I take for atrial fibrillation to slow my heart rate and keep that under control. About three days into that week, I was taking deep naps every afternoon because the Phenobarbital was making me sleepy. Paula was pretty mellow because her heart rate was a little bit slower than usual. I figured that out and switched them back and all was fine.

I was having a little trouble.

Another time, I accidentally doubled up one of her anti-seizure drugs. She started having issues like lethargy, balance issues, and bad double vision. I was wondering what was going on. I figured that it had to be drug-related because it came on all of a sudden. I got out the fact sheets that come with prescriptions and read through them for side effects. There was one that said that sure signs of an overdose are X, Y, and Z. I said to myself, "Well heck, she seems to have an overdose of that."

I looked in the pill container and sure enough, the dosage of the pill was two hundred milligrams and her dosage was two hundred milligrams twice a day. Inadvertently, I guess I was distracted by something and put two pills in both the morning and night slots, so she was doubling up on her dose.

I called the neurologist in Ohio who had given us his home phone number—the one Paula calls her druggie because he keeps her on an even keel with proper prescriptions. I was very concerned because one of the problems with an overdose of that particular drug is kidney failure. He suggested watching her for a day or two and going to get a kidney test in two days.

Luckily, nothing happened, but going on with life we had to learn to manage medications. We got bonus points from all our doctors for compliance because they said a lot of people don't take the drugs. Maybe they don't like the side effects, but I would encourage people to talk to your doctor. They want you to feel good; and to be safe and healthy.

One of the best things a person can do is pay attention to and follow their medication schedules. The doctors prescribe those drugs for a reason based on their training and experience, but it's up to us to follow their advice.

# CHAPTER 20

# CREATING A NEW LIFE & THE "NEW NORMAL"

We got the house mostly finished in 2010, moved in, and I took a big sigh of relief. It wasn't 100 percent done like Paula wanted. Really, it still isn't, but done is a four-letter word. We're living in it and loving it. Stuff will get done, or it won't. We're moving on to things that are more important and working on the remaining house things when we can.

We have settled nicely into the community here. Paula hits the road every day that it's possible, based on the weather. She has two four-wheel outdoor mobility scooters. They are her lifeline because they let her get out of the house and into the neighborhood (and into more trouble).

Her mobility scooters are important because she can't just be in the house. What we've done as much as we can is try to build as much activity and normal life into what is no longer a normal life. You have to redefine normal.

I don't focus on myself. When they were building the house, I wondered what I could do, so I created paths that go down through our woods. I even moved some small tree trunk pieces to the downhill side of the trails so I could level them out.

You can see a path down there that bends around a tree and comes up. There was a big tree that I was trying to cut through, and I couldn't cut, so I yelled up at the house, "Can you do me a favor?" A guy came and I asked him to move the trees, and poof, they were gone! I thanked him and continued on, but it was an incline and I had to level it out. Doug would say not to do that because it was not safe.

Sometime after we finished the house and most of the outside work, a friend of ours who founded a therapeutic riding center here in Brevard came to me and asked if I would be interested in serving on their board. I said yes. I really don't go into anything halfway, so I became the chair of the board and the de facto executive director. I spent a lot of time on this really important work. Paula sometimes gets jealous of the time I spend on this, but Free Rein Center serves a lot of people who get great benefits from their participation - participants and volunteers alike, so I'm happy to do it.

I tried to get Paula to ride there several times, but she is unwilling to do it if she has to have a horse leader and side walker again. She yearns to be able to get on a horse and just take off on an independent trail ride. The thought of riding in a ring, with assistants, is actually more of a negative thing than it is positive, it just reinforces her limitations.

As we've gone on with life, we've gotten even more involved with the community. We have a little community center up here. We love going to all the potlucks and keeping the roads clear of litter with roadside trash pickups. Paula greatly enjoys talking with everybody. She runs out of time before she runs out of people to talk to

We've gone to a lot of musical performances around town and have really gotten into the local music scene. Now we have our favorite bands that we try to go listen to whenever we can.

Paula is very much into yard work. She gets out on her outdoor scooter and does all sorts of things around the yard; planting, pulling weeds, and making trails through the woods.

There continues to be a struggle to balance and negotiate between what she wants to do and what I think is safe and therapeutic. For instance, when she was making trails through the woods, I made sure she had a phone with her. We have cordless phones that have intercoms, so if she got into a sticky situation or fell over, which she has done, she can call me and I can go down and help. It goes against my nature because I like to be there to make sure of her safety and security, but that's not good either. Paula started another round of physical and occupational therapy in 2014. We like to go back periodically to see what else we can do to help her continue improving.

When I went for the initial evaluation, the occupational therapist asked me, "Okay, what do you want to do?" In my most serious tone, I said, "I want to be able to use a chainsaw." He was very professional and wrote it down, but I knew it really shocked him. At my next visit, I told him I wasn't totally serious about the chainsaw (I was, really) but that I did want to be able to use my right arm and hand to do a lot more. I get upset because I can't do a lot of things I want to do. A lot of them aren't very high on Doug's priority list since he's got so much other stuff to do.

That's the fundamental conflict, and probably always will be. Paula gets frustrated at me because I tell her she can't do something or we don't need to do it right now. She wanted to go down Becky Mountain Road to visit some ladies that she likes down that way, but it's a steep, twisty mountain road. I told her, "If I catch you going down there, I'm going to take the batteries out of your cart and bury them in the backyard." End of story.

Before, you told me, "You don't wanna go down there." I thought, I've been down there. I went two or three times.

Just because you did something and survived it once doesn't mean it's a safe thing to do. That's an example of one of our more typical conflicts, and we're always going to have them. I'm quite sure that if the shoe was on the other foot and I had suffered the same injury, Paula would be able to tell the same story. She might not have been contracting to build the house, but we would be having the same conflicts about what's safe and therapeutic and I'd be the one complaining that she wouldn't let me do this or that and she'd be telling me not to do this.

I have been feeling worse because I want to do more, but he is doing more within the town and is more involved; back to a more normal life. I want to do stuff and I can't do it. I'm upset because I can't do them. I'm upset that Doug won't do what I want to do, those things that I would have done if I was normal.

I think that part of Paula resents me having to do things. It's related to that continuing struggle of who sees what as safe to do. Paula still has a few things going on that make it challenging for me: one of them is what I refer to as, "The bright shiny penny effect."

It's like the dog in the movie *Up*, whenever you're in the middle of something, the dog will holler, "Squirrel!" And then he's off—that's the bright shiny penny effect. She sees a lot of things she wants done, and for that period of time, it's the most important thing in the world and I need to attend to it.

I think of what I want to get done and tell Doug about it. I don't remember that I've told him before and it frustrates him too. He claims that I've told him six-eight things I want him to do on the short drive from our place into town. He's probably right, I just don't remember that I've told him and it's important to me at that point in time.

After a list of ten priorities in a week, I shut down and I can't attend to any of them. I wait and put things aside and if a particular task comes up often enough, I know I'd better do it. It's a coping mechanism on my part. Painting the last four windowsills in the house isn't quite as important as doing some other things I think I need to do.

I was used to being able to weed and I couldn't do it, so he should do it.

To this day, Paula's got a long list of things that she thinks I should be doing. I can't prioritize them, so I can't get to them. The honey do list has changed. Her mentality now is that she resents that I can't do it, or won't do it, because it's not a priority for me.

I think I've diagnosed myself with an emotional or neurological condition called executive function overload disorder. The part of your brain that performs executive functions, like planning, gets overloaded and doesn't function properly. When Paula starts telling me about all the things she wants me to do, I shut down because I can't process it all, so I just go to a different place. She resents that now. In many ways, the better she gets, the harder it is because she is somewhat more demanding, but that's okay.

He won't let me get someone to do stuff. I ask, "Can we hire someone to do it?" But he says, "Oh, we don't need to spend money on that. I'll do it."

I'm thinking that some of the things she wants to get done aren't important enough to spend money on right now; it's not that it's not important at all. I think that the bright shiny penny effect is a result of her head injury. That, plus the fact that she would just go do things before the injury that she really can't do now. When Paula sees something that she thinks is important, it's the most important thing in the whole world right then. She's very focused until she sees the next thing that she thinks needs to be done.

The bright shiny penny effect is also a challenge for me because I can't shift gears as easily as she does. I've got a lot going on at home, in the community, and with Free Rein. Arguably, you could say that I'm not being smart by devoting time and attention to Free Rein, but it really is an outlet for my creative and organizational skills and interests. It's also a way for me to make positive contributions to the community to which I feel so strongly attached. I like being involved in things where we're making something good happen.

Everybody else gets to see the positive side of me, but Doug gets stuck with the bitching side. I don't think we had that problem when I was normal because I could do things; if I wanted to have it done, I could do it. Now I can't do many things. It may be that my brain has gotten better, so I get more upset that I can't do things.

But I'm evil, because I do things and I'm just irritating. In Ohio, you know, Doug said, don't get up out of your chair, but when he was at work, I thought I could use the vacuum cleaner from the chair and so I vacuumed the house. The scooter was too hard, so I was standing up and pushing it. I would sit on the sofa and think about how I would have to get up, so I would scoot up by the arm and use the other arm to help me get up. I would figure out how to do things. I don't know if I ever told Doug that I got stuck in the barn in Ohio.

Or, I just try to do things and think, "Oh, I shouldn't have done that" afterwards. If something happens to me, it's not a shock, it's just, "Oh well, it happened." I remember yelling, "Doug, come down," when I'd fall over up here and, "Hey Doug, can you get me out?"

When I'm stuck in the scooter. I don't whine. I'm ornery and stubborn. I don't remember being like that when I was normal, though. That's probably because I could do just about anything I wanted to do then.

Before her injury, if she got angry at me for not doing something, she'd just go do it. Now she gets angry at me because something she wants to do is not high in my priorities. When I tell her I can't do that thing right now, she gets upset. I get upset when I feel she wants me to do something right now that, to me, isn't nearly as important as something else I need to do. Sometimes, I tell her that she is focusing too much on doing something and not on getting something done. I don't have a lot of extra time to do something that I don't see as accomplishing some higher priority thing, even though I know it's important to her.

Doug did a great job of getting ready to build the house, building it, and getting us moved in. Then his focus shifted to doing other stuff and not all the things I wanted to get done. Before my accident, I'd paint and do lots of other stuff, and I'd do all that. We still have a few doors and window frames that aren't painted yet.

Yes, we still have a couple of window frames that aren't painted yet. And we've been in the house for more than five years.

# CHAPTER 21

# LIVING TOGETHER & BUILDING A NEW RELATIONSHIP

In many ways, the better Paula gets, the more challenging it is for me as her companion and caregiver. She is expanding her horizons (and has been for the last thirteen years) and has more things that she wants to do and have done. She wants to hire people to come and do yard work and clear out the woods, something that she can't do that she would've done otherwise.

There is a perverse saying that I read or heard during that first year after her injury—it might have been in Living with Brain Injury, or it might have been from a support group. It was, "How do you grieve for somebody who has not died?"

Paula is not the same person that I married and grew up

with. The year 2015 was interesting because it marks the point in time when one-third of our married life has been post-injury.

Even though it seems like the accident was just yesterday, that event defines a greater part of our marriage and our life together as time goes on. This is very sobering to me every year.

We are still learning the thriving part of life, what life is all about, what we can do and what we can't do, what we have time to do and what we don't. The hard part of the survival and driving mode, the recovery phase, is that this isn't the same person you spent all those years with.

A challenge as Paula's spouse, but it could work the same as with a son or a daughter, is that you get really good at being a caregiver and you lose focus on being a companion. Those are two separate things. That's something that I still struggle with, because when the loved one survives and you run this rigid schedule of therapy and recovery, they can become more of a patient to you.

For the first two-thirds of our life together, we both worked and we didn't spend twenty-four hours a day together. I don't care how much you love your soul mate; the person you're made for, spending 24/7 together is too much time to spend together. You have to be honest about that.

I have only taken a couple of breaks in caregiving. The football team from the college where I taught has been a perennial playoff team in Division III, and they generally always go to the Stagg Bowl which is the Division III championship game in Salem, Virginia. They went to the championship game all but one of the ten years I was teaching at Mount Union and I never went. They've been every year since I left, too. We're actually closer to Salem now than we were in Ohio, so I've gone twice since we moved to North Carolina.

The first year, a friend of ours stayed with Paula in the house. Driving up to Virginia knowing I was going to be gone overnight for the very first time was very different than driving to the store to get groceries.

That was the first time I'd been away from Paula overnight except when she was in the hospital or in rehab, and it was twelve years after the accident. It was probably too long a time to wait to take a break, but it was self-imposed. I didn't trust anybody to be with her because we had invested too much. I'm not comfortable with her being home alone overnight yet.

Driving up to Virginia that first time, I was thinking less about enjoying the game and wondering more about if Paula was okay. I think I called twice on the way up. It worked out fine, at least from what I heard.

Another challenge we have is a lack of conversation. We've been married thirty-nine years and I'm convinced that at a certain point in marriage you've talked about all the stuff you need to really talk about on a daily basis. I'm sure that we would probably have the same concerns as many couples who have been married a long time if Paula had not had her head injury that, but her injury and subsequent limitations in ability to do things she wants to do probably bring them into a sharper focus.

I'm convinced that this is part of the difference between men and women. I'm not trying to sound sexist here, but I probably end up sounding that way. It is not my intent. Women like to talk things out, and guys like to fix problems. Problem solved? I'm happy. If my wife has a problem, she'll talk about it for a while and then she's happy. Did we fix it? I don't know, but we're happy!

Our situation has brought more focus on that typical issue between longer-term married people because Paula doesn't have other people to talk to, at least in her mind. She calls friends and family every day. When we go out somewhere, whether it's to the store or out to eat, she talks to everybody she runs into. She meets no strangers, as they say. As a consequence of being together round the clock, we do need some alone time.

But we're not together a whole lot. In the morning, Doug gets his cereal and goes into his office to do our banking stuff, check email, look at Facebook, work on Free Rein or See Off Mountain community activities, and watch the news (which I really don't like to watch). He cooks dinner while we watch the evening news. At night, we watch some of our favorite TV shows or watch a movie. We don't sit around and talk much. I don't go out with other people. I normally go in the car with Doug wherever we need or want to go.

We eat together. We go out to drive to therapy and to shop, but we don't sit around and just talk about stuff much. Paula really doesn't like talking about news, financial things, and current events. All those things bother or scare her. I like talking about current events and politics. She loves to watch old movies and I don't, so that isn't a good topic of conversation for us either.

It doesn't bother me that she doesn't want to watch the news, but I go into my room and watch the news. That makes it worse because the things that I want to talk about, Paula doesn't want to talk about. It's fairly typical amongst couples, but this brings it in to sharper focus.

I was probably too focused on her recovery and less focused on if she wanted to go and get ice cream, although we tried to do that. We would go out to the movies and stuff. My principle focus became caregiving because that's the most important thing that was going on. It's still a continuing struggle to balance that caregiver versus the nurturing, loving companion role. It's an internal struggle that we each deal with in different ways. It's not easy to talk about... and even harder to do something to change.

He sees me broken and he sees what he can do to fix it. I think about what I can do, not about what I've done, just about what I can do.

Caregiving all comes down to managing your time and stress, and sometimes that means getting out and doing something different. I used to read books, six or seven a year. I don't make time to read books now, and that troubles me. If I invest the time in reading that book it means I can't be doing something else.

I've given up a lot, and part of it is a matter of time. I'm much more careful now about my safety and health so I can continue to be around for Paula. I gave up downhill skiing; I sold my skis and boots when we moved from Ohio because if I got hurt or went offline for a little bit, it would be a real problem. I like to play golf. When I was in the navy I used to play golf two or three times a week and I was pretty good. Over the last ten years, I've probably averaged playing three times a year.

My body's gotten older, too. My Uncle Arthur (arthritis) moved into my spine a few years ago. I worked hard on the house and that had an impact on my shoulders, so I can't do some of the things I used to do. I used to play a lot of softball, and there are over sixty leagues I could get into, but I haven't because I hurt more after I play now.

Doug has been through a hell of a lot of stuff. I think back on how he's been working so hard on keeping me going and how many times he has to pick me up. We wonder why his back is sore. He spends a lot of time at the computer doing Free Rein this and that, and I feel that he needs a different kind of exercise. The computer is not exercise to me.

Like a lot of people in the world now, I probably spend more time in front of my computer screen than I should. Sometimes I feel dumb about spending time on Facebook or playing games, but it's an opportunity to just put my mind at idle and just go slow.

I need to work on that balance of not being on the computer so much and maybe painting a windowsill from time to time. I've never really been much of an exerciser. I don't go to the gym, nor have I ever been one to do what might be called structured exercise. I walk around a lot and maintain the yard and the house, so I'm in pretty good shape for my age.

When I was in the navy, I did the physical fitness test that was required twice a year and that was pretty much it. I participated in several sports: golf, softball, and volleyball. I went skiing and swam when those activities were available nearby, but I didn't go to a pool just to swim laps. I'm not somebody that you're ever gonna see with a FitBit on my arm.

Paula has always been extremely active. She still is, but now she's a lot more mentally active than physically active because she can't do a lot of the things she used to do. Before her injury, it was common to find Paula out in the woods with a chainsaw and a *Walkman* cutting down brush and trees with a tank full of gas, and then resting for a little bit before burning it.

Paula hasn't given up her image of herself, which is a great thing because she's more the person she used to be than ever and will continue to get to be more of that person. Paula has another unique trait. She remembers something from her early days that a therapist did that was specifically designed to help her do something to get her along to another level. She wants to go back and do that thing again, and we discuss this a lot. I say, "You know that was designed to help you do this, which you have mastered and don't need to do anymore." I think this is because she understood what those earlier activities were designed to do, but has trouble figuring out what would be required now.

Early on, we worked her on a *Total Gym*, doing leg thrusts. That was required to get the muscles of her upper leg fired up and communicating with her brain again. After she got that going, it became more important to work on her lower leg and ankle, so we would do that. She kept wanting to go back and work on the upper leg muscles too, but I'd say, "You have those and they're getting better on their own; we need to work on things that aren't working well yet."

Paula's the least complacent person I've ever met because she's always looking for something to do to move forward and do better. This is partially because she has never been an inactive person.

Understanding the progression of activity and therapies and that sort of stuff in her life is important. It doesn't do a lot of good to go back and repeat things that you don't need to do anymore. It's more important to always be looking for the next thing that you need to do.

We have a platform walker downstairs because there's a chance Paula's going to need it again at some point in the future. She needed it again for a short time when she broke her leg some ten years after her injury. She was moving a pile of wood from one side of the basement to the other, even though it was still a pile of wood and you could still see it. In the process, she fell out of the rolling office chair she was using and broke both the lower leg bones (tibia and fibula) in her right leg. She had to have a rod put in the tibia and was not able to bear any weight on that leg for six weeks. This was a good example of her confusing doing something with getting something done, from my perspective. She did something she wanted to do, but it didn't really accomplish much... and introduced a good deal of risk into her life.

I was in the basement straightening up a pile of wood when I fell. I called up to Doug to come down because I thought I just broke my leg. When he came down, I was leaning against the wall. He checked things out and got me back into the chair. I told him he could help me get back into my scooter outside so I could go up and get in the car to go to the hospital. He said no way and that he was calling an ambulance. I cried about needing an ambulance. Doug drove to the hospital and was waiting for me in the emergency room when I got out of the ambulance. I had to have surgery the next morning. Free Rein's gala fundraising event was that night and Doug was the chair of the board. He said that he'd stay there with me instead of going, but I made him leave and go to the gala.

The reason I hurt myself is probably that I'm a clean freak. Doug is not a clean freak. Another time, back when we were still in Ohio, there was a small tack room that had all the feed and stuff in the barn and I was tidying it up. I was standing up, and then I turned around and fell. So I had to call a neighbor to help get me up. I don't remember if I was on the floor or not, but I had moved myself up to sitting on bags. The neighbor girl wasn't strong enough to get me up so I told her to give me some pressure and then I moved over to another thing at a higher level, and so on, and I was able to get up. I handled it.

Paula has a habit of not telling me about things like this that she thinks I might not be happy hearing. This was one of many things like it that I never heard about until she started telling her stories when we started writing this book. Neither of those were life-threatening things, only speed bumps in the road to recovery. When she fell out of the chair and broke her leg, it snapped us from the thrive phase of our life back into the drive phase, because Paula was non-weight bearing for six to eight weeks and it impacted everything we had to do. She needed a lot more help going to the bathroom again. We just recalibrated and asked ourselves what we needed to do to recover from that and get back to thriving.

One of the ongoing limitations that Paula has is the ability to prioritize and understand the relationship between decisions and outcomes. She will disagree with this and I understand that, but with all head injuries, whether it's a stroke or a traumatic brain injury, you end up with some limitations. Some of them are physical and some are cognitive or mental. Some are very minor and some of them are very important.

Paula has struggled and pushed through a lot of the physical and cognitive limitations, but she confuses doing something with getting something done. Activity is not the same as accomplishment. I will find her doing things that, in my mind, have absolutely no long-term benefit, like moving boxes from one shelf to another shelf. There's still stuff in boxes, but now the boxes are on a different shelf. There are a lot of examples like that, and part of that is a difference in priorities, too.

We also have to be careful that Paula doesn't get overly tired.

When I first started out going to places again, I would go somewhere and visit and then I'd go and lie on the sofa and sleep for a while, or lay in the bedroom and sleep. Now, I have to be careful that I don't stay too long with larger groups of people because I get screwy on talking.

In busy places or in large crowds, sensory overload kicks in. Too much stimulus gets to her and causes her to start to shut down. It may actually increase the chances of her having a seizure, so I watch this very carefully. I've learned some of Paula's seizure triggers and what's a good thing to do and what's not a good thing to do. Paula doesn't need to sleep as much now. She may take an afternoon nap five days out of the week, particularly when she's in therapy. She's in back-to-back physical and occupational therapy now, so we have to build in some recovery time for that. That wears her out. She comes home and may sleep for two hours because they work her pretty hard, but it's important work.

My brain gets working and it doesn't feel like I'm doing anything, but then I come home and I have to sleep.

She's physically and emotionally tired.

I don't ride horses anymore. Doug works at Free Rein, and theoretically I could go down and ride, but I don't want to ride because I would have to have people there to help.

We've talked about that a number of times since we've lived here. Paula could obviously go ride at Free Rein or any other therapeutic riding facility, but in her case, it would actually be negative now. As she's improved, she feels more like her old self. Her self-image of riding a horse is leaping up into the saddle and trundling off through the woods for several hours on her own, and she can't do that now. She thinks she can and she wants to. If she could do that, she would love to. Heck, if she could do that again, we'd probably buy a piece of land and have a horse again.

I have very vivid dreams. In one dream, we drove up and there was a barn where they have therapy horses. People helped me get on the horse and then let me ride. And I rode from the barn down to the house.

She still likes being around horses, and when we go down to Free Rein, she goes out in the barn and talks to all the horses, because she's a horse whisperer. The idea of getting on a horse and not being in control is bad for her emotionally. She would not want to have a side walker or a horse leader, but she's been off horses for so long that she would have to go back through that progression.

I'm also more concerned about money and there would be money involved for me having to learn the stuff again. Doug tells me that we're doing fine, but I don't want to spend the money. I just want to ride on trails in the woods. When I was at Pegasus Farm, the place in Ohio, they'd let me ride on the outdoor trails every so often. I'd have a leader and two people following (including Doug). We'd walk through puddles and I didn't give a hoot about them.

Paula thought that was great fun when we had to walk through the mud puddles and mosquitoes. She was out in the woods on a horse, and that's pure heaven to her. She thinks that she wouldn't have to go through that progression back to where she was as a rider, but as the chair of the board of Free Rein (not as her husband); I wouldn't let her ride without going through that progression. It's a matter of risk management and proper protocol.

Another thing that we continue to disagree on, and sometimes argue about, is that Paula has a Medic Alert tag on her necklace that she absolutely hates wearing. It's for TBI survivors and seizure disorder. She's still at risk even though life is going pretty well. I feel that it is very important for her to wear it so folks would know what was going on if she had a seizure again and I wasn't there to help.

I still do take more risks than he is comfortable with. I wanted to ride the riding mower, but I couldn't take that risk. I didn't ever fool with the mower because Doug wouldn't let me, but I was ticked off because I wanted to. The yard that we had in Ohio was totally flat and the trees that we had were big enough so I wouldn't crash. I wouldn't "bonk" into the fence, either. I figured that it would be something that I could do, but he was too scared for me. He let me do it once, but insisted on walking along beside me. That defeated the whole reason I wanted to do it, so he could go do something else and I could help out more.

I'm ornery. If I'm going up a hill in the scooter and it's tough, I'll put my foot out and help push it. Doug says, "Don't do that. Keep your foot up and don't ever touch the ground." Sometimes Doug goes into a panic about me doing something. Other times, I do things and sometimes I have to call him: "Hey Doug, I'm stuck." I look very carefully at the woods before I go to make sure there are no stumps or anything. Even so, I sometimes have to call him and ask him to come get me unstuck. I hate that.

I was rolling down our road in my four wheel scooter and not paying attention to where the road bends and there's a little dip in the road, so I tipped over. There was a guy cleaning up the porta-potty there. I said, "Hi! Can you do me a favor?" He came up and said yes. "Can you help me up?" He picked my scooter and me up and I went on my way.

Another challenge for me is that Paula seems to want to control a lot of things she doesn't need to. I suppose that she has so little control over so much of her life after the injury that she just tries to control many things that she isn't even directly involved in. This manifests itself in her telling me which pot to use to cook something in, whether to call or email someone I want to get in touch with, and a host of other such things. It also shows up much more post-injury when she tries to tell her friends and family what to do. I don't remember her doing this before her injury. I try to tell her that many people don't like being told what they should do and that it might alienate some of them, but it's become a habit of sorts.

# CHAPTER 22

# BLENDING LIFE WITH CONTINUED IMPROVEMENTS, HOWEVER SMALL

Paula is still improving, and continuing to drive forward, many years after the accident. Why? Because she's still working toward making improvements. We get her back into therapy every couple of years to see what else she can do, and what we should be doing to get her a little more capability to do things to improve her physical strength and muscle control. She started another round of physical and occupational therapy thirteen years after the injury. Her gait and balance still weren't good, so we wanted to focus on those specific things.

She has recently graduated to a new ankle-foot orthotic that makes her use the muscles in her ankle and foot more. After a few sessions in this new round of therapy, she gained the ability to walk on the treadmill for short periods of time without her ankle foot orthotic at all, under the close supervision of her physical therapist. This was much more in our minds than just another step forward, if you'll pardon the pun.

When I go to therapy, I have sixty minutes to work with them and then I come home and it seems like Doug doesn't do many of the exercises with me. That upsets me. I know that some of them are hard on him and his body, but I'd like to do more. In therapy, they had me walking without the brace for short periods of time.

Before my accident, I bent my knee when I walked. Afterwards, I wasn't and the way I walked wasn't correct. The therapists are trying to fix the way I walk so I'm not screwing my knees up because I've probably done some of that. I have gotten a new ankle brace that makes me do more of the work of walking, so that's good.

I also work with an occupational therapist who's working with my hand; he works more with the brain trying to get my hand and brain to get together. I have to tell my brain and my hand together to go this way or that way. I told him, "Yell at me and tell me to do it because I like to get pushed hard." He and I do an exercise where we cross hands and I pull him toward me and he pulls me back. I told him, "I like that more, because I'm gonna win."

When we went into therapy the last time, they recommended a cane, so now she walks with a cane and it's much better. The injury has created new risks and problems even though she's recovered a lot of strength, flexibility, balance, and cognitive ability.

She still has lingering deficits in all those areas because not all those systems have been rewired yet. I'm convinced the proverbial electricians are still up there working, but they're working slowly. Some things may never get reconnected, but we're confident that some still can be. A lot of it is attitude. If you feel like you've gotten to where you're going, you've probably gotten to where you're going. If you think there's still room to grow, then you'll probably keep growing.

Paula challenges her therapists: "Hey, you're not being tough enough on me!" They look at her funny, and then they do push. We refer to physical therapists as physical terrorists but in a lighthearted way. Their job is to push you and maybe let you cry a little bit, but say, "Okay, get back up. Do it." If you're not going to do that, you're not going to get out of it as much as you can, and you won't regain as much as you could.

A lot of doctors, caregivers, and therapists will tell you that you regain most of what you'll regain in a year, and then plateau. In our experience, the gains and regaining of abilities certainly slows down, but we are thirteen years out and Paula's still making gains. All the body systems, balance, strength, cognitive functions, sight, and speech, are all still improving at their own speeds. Sometimes one will stop for a while and sometimes it won't.

We have friends who come to visit once or twice a year and when they leave, they take me aside and tell me, "You know, Paula's really continuing to do better." I may not have even realized it, because the small, incremental improvements are harder for me to see. Living together 24/7, I don't notice a lot of the changes. It's the old frog and the pan of water analogy: If you put a frog in a pan of cold water and slowly turn up the heat, you can literally boil it to death. It doesn't feel the changes in temperature because it happens so slowly. There's always hope for more improvement.

The drive to recover has become more blended with actually living, and we mixed continuing to recover into trying to insert more normal things into our lives. While we were going through therapy and driving to recover some basic stuff, we'd go see movies and go out to dinner. We'd go visit friends.

The progression was goal-oriented in my mind. The first goal was to survive what happened, and the second one is to recover as much as possible. The third, thriving, you have to sneak in there, because if you're not careful, you'll always be driving to recover and you'll forget about living. You have to do both. In retrospect, getting on with living helps you recover more, too.

I spend some time thinking about how we can make our life even better and more enjoyable. Complacency is something everybody suffers from. People that are born and raised in one place or live in a place for a long time get complacent about doing the things that they should be out doing and seeing.

You think you'll get around to it because you live there. In our experience in the navy, we would move someplace and know we were only going to be there for three years and we got really good at exploring and learning about new places fairly quickly. Within six or eight weeks, we would have done more than many people who were born and raised there had.

For example, we got orders to Lakehurst, New Jersey, fairly close to Ellis Island. I've always wanted to see the Statue of Liberty and Ellis Island, so our third week there we drove up to Ellis Island and the Statue of Liberty. It was a busy Saturday with a big long line, and I'm standing behind a guy in line that's about my age, and I said, "You know, I've always wanted to come here." He said, "Yeah, me too." I asked him where he was from and he turned around and pointed to the shore and said, "You see the house with the green roof, second row in? I was born and raised there." I said, "And you've never been here?!" That was just galvanizing to me. Oddly enough, I fell into the same trap. I was teaching in Alliance, Ohio, fifteen miles from the Pro Football Hall of Fame. I'm an avid football fan, yet the whole ten years I was there, I never went and I still haven't been to the Pro Football Hall of Fame.

We need to get back to something we used to do before her injury. Once a year, if not more often, we'd pick a couple of days or even a whole week and think, "We just moved here, so what do we need to do or go see?" It's hard to do that, especially once you get into routines. I'm working with Free Rein, Paula's in therapy again, and there are many things we're involved in here. We've lived here full time for six years now and there are so many things we need to still do. The complacency of thinking we'll get around to it can keep us from thriving as much as we might.

That word complacency applies not just to getting on with normal life, but the whole process, from surviving to driving to thriving. Early on, in the survival mode, you could be complacent by saying, "The doctor's got this. I just need to listen." But that's not true. You have to be an active participant in the survival mode and in the recovery. You can't be complacent. If you see something the therapist is or isn't doing that you like or don't like, then you must say something.

# CHAPTER 23

# SUMMING UP & SOME THINGS WE'D HAVE DONE DIFFERENTLY

There are a lot of things that I might have done differently at the scene of the original accident if I had thought about it, like using that big cornfield close to where Paula fell off for a helicopter landing, for instance. I could have said, "Get a helicopter in here, NOW!" But I figured I'd leave it to the experts. They know what to do, they know where they are, and they know where she needs to go. They are the experts. Next time I'll know, but I don't want to have a next time.

I almost wish we had bought the donkey that morning because we would have been bringing the donkey home at two in the afternoon instead of being on horseback in the woods.

But you can't go back and change the past. It does absolutely no good to second-guess yourself looking backwards. There were fifteen decisions that day that, had they had slightly different outcomes, would have resulted in no accident in the first place, or her death in the worst case scenario. Once you start that, there is just no stopping it as there is such a long line of prior decisions you have to work back through.

When this happened, we didn't have our cell phone with us. We were lucky that the kids in the woods had a cell phone with them. Now, I would never leave the house without my cell phone, not because I use it a lot, but because it's too important to not have the capability to get in touch with someone immediately in case of an emergency.

To the extent that it's possible, I recommend finding the best in-patient rehab center that you can and going there because this is an investment in the rest of your life. You can't just go to the local rehab facility or nursing home closest to home or the hospital because they may not be the best environment. There may be a great rehab center right next to your hospital, but shop around and talk to the experts. Find out where in the world you need to take your loved one and get them there.

If it means that they go there alone for six months, know that the staff at a good place can take good care of them. If the rehab facility near my sister's house in Monroeville hadn't been there, or not been as highly regarded, we probably would've taken Paula to Denver or Houston. I might not have been able to be there the whole time; I might have only been able to go for four days a month, but I would've done that because that's what it takes.

The night of Paula's accident, I came home and sent out an email to a bunch of friends. It was just informational, telling them about what had happened and what was going on right then. I asked them to send prayers, positive thoughts, karma, or whatever floated their particular boat. I needed more positive energy in the room with her. They responded very well. It was helpful and cathartic to me to come home after I visited with Paula over the next weeks and months and be able to pour out my feelings and share a status or updates with others.

There was nobody else at home to share with, so getting connected to family and friends was important. I talked to people on the cell phone until the battery ran dry every day. Now, there are online communities like CaringBridge where you can post the initial story about your loved one and then post the updates. People subscribe to it and follow your story. I would definitely recommend opening up a CaringBridge account where your friends and family can keep track of your loved one. Since then, I've had friends who were experiencing personal tragedies. I was on their CaringBridge pages often, trying to give them whatever support and help that I could.

A very real problem I had when Paula came home from rehab was having enough refrigerator and freezer space for all the food that people would bring over unsolicited. After about five days, I put out a note that said, "We have enough food for six years, so I'll let you know if I need anything, but thanks a lot!"

In Paula's case, one of the best things people could do is just come and spend time with her and talk to her. An old friend coming to talk for an hour and a half is awesome because it's rekindling memories, it's great therapy - both cognitive and emotional. People can really help in that way. I encourage people to visit and don't bring food; just come and spend an hour. If the person that's recovering falls asleep, then they can either wait or go home, but they will have made a real positive contribution by just showing up.

We became very appreciative of each and every one of our caregivers and medical providers; the doctors, the therapists, and the nurses. As Paula was recovering, people made comments to me like, "You're such an amazing person dealing with all of this," and I'd say, "No, I'm like a farmer. I can plow the ground, plant the seed, and hope for rain, but Paula is that seed."

The other thing I found was that people assumed that I was, somehow, special for sticking around and helping Paula throughout this long, strange journey. That sort of bothered me, as I think a lot of people do the same thing and people outside their immediate circle of friends and family never hear about it. I don't feel like I did anything special, just what I promised to do on the day we were married.

I think that a small minority of people who do otherwise get a lot of publicity because bad news seems to sell better than good news. Others, focusing on the bad news story, assume that a majority of people do the same. They are the ones people tell stories about and those negative stories spread more rapidly and widely than do stories like ours.

If Paula didn't have the drive and the desire to get better, she wouldn't have. To a large extent, all her doctors, her therapists, and nurses were in the same boat. We are enablers, but she's the one doing the work. Never lose focus on the fact that the patient is the person that's got to do the work. If they aren't doing it, then you've got to help them want to do it, because if they don't want to do it, it's not going to happen. You can put all the things in place, but it's just not going to happen without the motivation to survive, drive, and thrive.

We really do appreciate all those people who helped her,

like her neurosurgeon and neurologist. They are high-powered folks. They're some of the most highly trained specialists in the world, and I had never met one before this. What I'd heard was that they could have a god complex or aloof personalities.

What we saw was very different, at least in Dr. Markarian and Dr. Al Jaberi. While we still lived in Ohio, we'd take Dr. Markarian a bottle of good red wine and a box of good chocolates every year at Christmas just to thank him. Several times, we went to his office and he'd be there working with patients. We'd intend just to drop a gift off at the nurses' station for him, but the nurses would go back and tell him we were there, and he'd come sit in the conference room with us for fifteen-twenty minutes. He actually set his patients aside for a time to sit and talk with us.

Every time that we talked to him, he would disclose more about her injury. It turns out that she had a half-inch hole in one of the main veins that returns blood to the body, and that blood is toxic to brain cells. That's why part of her left temporal lobe was dead and had to be removed. When we were in the conference room he said, "You cost me a dinner!" We asked him what he meant, and he said, "Well, when I opened her skull, blood flew all over the operating room and soaked the anesthesiologist and he made me take him out to dinner."

It was three or four years after the accident before we heard that one. Now, that is merely interesting. Then, it was pretty shocking. Paula and I still keep in touch with some of her former doctors and some of her former therapists.

A few years ago, my aunt died in Pittsburgh. We wanted to go through Ohio and visit with some folks. Paula made one of her Untamed Horse sculptures for Dr. Al Jaberi, her neurologist who lived there. We contacted him, saying, "We're going to be in Ohio these two nights. We'd like to take you and your wife out for dinner one night when we're there."

He said they'd be happy to go, so this busy, high-powered neurologist met us for dinner at 5:00 and brought his wife, who was the chief medical officer at a local hospital. She stayed through dinner but had to leave to pick up their son. But Dr. Al Jaberi stayed. We started dinner at five and left at nine; we just sat and talked for almost four hours.

The horse she gave him is named Omari, which means friendship in Syrian. Dr. Al Jaberi is from Aleppo, Syria. Paula gave him this horse and he was pretty touched by that.

One year after Paula came home, we threw a great big *thank you* party at our house in Ohio. We called it, "Thanksgiving in July." It was a picnic and we invited all the doctors, nurses, and therapists who had any contact with Paula since the afternoon of her injury.

We had about twenty people come from Monroeville, from Akron, and from Alliance. A group of folks from Monroeville carpooled over for the day. We made up an invitation to send to them that said, "We're thankful in July for what you've done to get us here and we want to throw this little picnic to honor you and show our love and thanks." It was a fun day.

Her speech therapist from HealthSouth, who hadn't seen her in over a year, came from Monroeville and was pretty impressed with the improvements Paula had made since they last saw one another.

One advantage of that day for us was the positive reinforcement: "You guys are doing important work and it really makes a big difference, so keep doing it." I'm guessing if we invited that network of people down here to Brevard, some of them would come down if they knew how beautiful it was. But maybe not all twenty of them.

If I could tell people with traumatic brain injuries one thing, it would be to stay positive. I'd encourage them to talk to people and tell them that this is the way you are now - deal with it! People who don't have a problem, or this bad of a problem, enjoy what they can do. The therapy helps me to stay positive. I can play around with people and I love that more than any of the therapy because I can harass them and talk to anybody I see. That's the way I am in stores. I talk to people and I always tell 'em to do as good as you can. It ain't worth it to waste time.

The images of the day of Paula's accident are still very vivid in my mind. They can start replaying themselves at the slightest provocation. Our lives changed dramatically in that instant when Paula slid off Clypso and hit the ground. It is amazing to me how far she has come since then. We are still learning about some of those changes and what they mean to each of us as a couple, and will continue to do so for a long time to come.

The memories of her accident, the initial survival phase, and the driving to recover phase are no less vivid in my mind, but they are less painful as we continue enjoying our lives in what we can only refer to as our new normal. I guess that means that we are, after all, successfully thriving. Paula and I wish you well if you are reading this book and have your own personal story of surviving, driving, and thriving, whatever part of that journey you may be in.

Please remember that it is a journey without a destination

if you continue to seek ways to thrive more effectively. That journey is called living a good life and we highly recommend it.

# AFTERWORD

## YOUR PERSPECTIVE DRIVES YOUR LIFE

Words and images by Paula Poad

There once was a very sad person who was sitting, looking at nothing... A unicorn came up to the person...

"Why are you so sad?" asked the unicorn. "I just feel sad... nothing to be happy for," sighed the person.

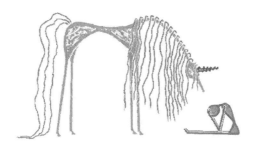

"Well, I love you," whispered the unicorn. The person looked up and saw the unicorn's heart and asked...

"That is good... but what should I be happy for?"

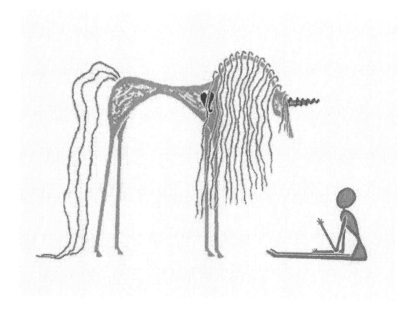

"Well," the unicorn said, "Look up to the sky and see the stars.

It shows that there are both good and bad. If you only see the bad and sad things in life, then it will be dark. You will always be looking at life that way. If you see the good and happy, the lovely and joyful, then, it'll be bright and you can look at life as good. Which do you want your life to be?"

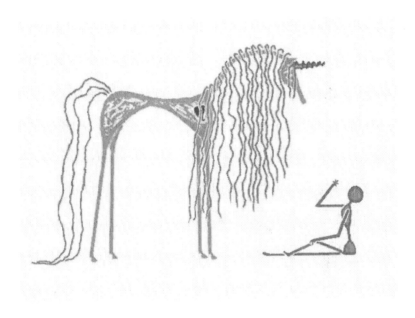

The person stood up, looked up into the sky, and saw a brightly shining star in the sky. The person touched the unicorn. On the inside, the person felt a joyful and happy heart beating.

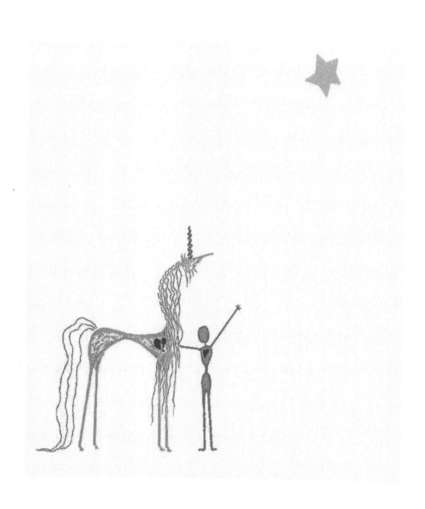

# Life is good!

70369023R00114

Made in the USA
Columbia, SC
05 May 2017